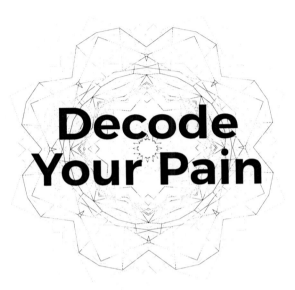

Decode Your Pain

Dr. Kevin Gyurina

Decode Your Pain

Copyright © 2017 Celebrity Expert Author
All Rights Reserved.
Unauthorized duplication or distribution is strictly prohibited.

ISBN-13: 978-0-9988546-2-5
ISBN-10: 0-9988546-2-X

Published by: Celebrity Expert Author
http://celebrityexpertauthor.com

Canadian Address:
1108 - 1155 The High Street,
Coquitlam, BC, Canada
V3B.7W4
Phone: (604) 941-3041
Fax: (604) 944-7993

US Address:
1300 Boblett Street
Unit A-218
Blaine, WA 98230
Phone: (866) 492-6623
Fax: (250) 493-6603

Table of Contents

Introduction

The All-Time Low. We've All Been There

If you've gone through rough times or you feel like you're stuck at a low point in some part of your life, don't worry. It happens to everyone and it's supposed to. Hitting rock bottom feels awful at the time but it's a necessary part of life. If you're there right now, I know how painful it can be. In fact, I'm going to share two of the lowest points in my life and how they have redirected me on the path to creating a life I love.

It's not always easy. We are so used to avoiding pain at all costs. We use distraction, numb ourselves with social media, food, drugs, and alcohol and ignore whole areas of our lives just to feel like we can cope. But just because you don't look at them, the things you don't like don't go away. Problems have a tendency to get bigger and bigger until you take care of them. And sometimes, as was the case with me quite literally, they have to blow up in your face before you take the necessary action to change your life.

2007, for all intents and purposes, should have been a high point of my life. I had recently graduated as a doctor of chiropractic and my life as a real person in the real world had just begun. I was sitting in a chiropractic seminar, listening to one of our industry leaders, Dr. James Chestnut, ask questions about health, beliefs and philosophies on life. My personal answers left me thoroughly disgusted with myself.

I was 27 years old, 70 pounds overweight, had high blood pressure, high cholesterol, was prediabetic, impotent and had signs of mouth cancer. How could I be a professional health practitioner, preaching the virtues of healthy living when my health was such a train wreck?

Only five years earlier at age 22 I had been at the peak of my health and now I was definitely in a deep, dark valley.

The Wake Up Call

At that moment I realized I had to do something. I needed to start practicing what I preached. I had to take control of my health, my nutrition, my exercising and my mind. And that's just what I did. In fact now, I'm rising to a new peak. At 36 I was in better shape than I was at age 22, and in various ways I continued to improve.

That was the start of my journey into the model of practice that I use with my patients now.

Maybe you've reached a point in your life where you realize that you've been slowly sliding downhill. Or perhaps you're having a wake up call moment right now, with a health scare, not liking what you see in the mirror, not being able to do what you used to do, or just being plain tired with your state of physical well-being.

Downward Momentum

Until that pivotal moment in 2007 I did not know that I had dipped down that far. When we get on a track, we tend to pick up speed and build momentum in one direction. Reaching my all time low had actually started many years earlier when I left home to go to school. I broke up a long-term relationship. I had gotten away from my upbringing. To cover up the pain I turned to video games, eating and alcohol.

At 22 I was playing college football and looked outwardly healthy but the downward momentum was building. I was eating massive amounts in the dining hall, I partied hard and I played hard. I was chewing tobacco on the bus with the teammates and was using alcohol and cigarettes to feel good in the moment during the weekends. When there was a problem in life I could always turn to that feeling and escape. That feeling turned on me. I had to do more and more of it to get the same feeling.

By the time I realized what I had done, I was fat and pre-diabetic with high blood pressure and mouth cancer. I was in a worse state than a lot of the people that come to see me for help! I had to stop this momentum before I could turn it around.

Building Upward Momentum

For the next few years, I would practice what I preached and I continually saw improvements in my health and well-being. Weight melted off of me, I began to exercise more and started having a muscular look. I stopped the tobacco at all levels, ate real food that was organic and pure and began to have positivity and motivation return in my life.

At age 32, I was in better shape than I was at 21 and continuing to improve.

But as life would have it, the path I was on needed some readjustment. This time it was not physical. It was more of a mental shift and life-changing turning point. I realized through a series of business decisions and practices, that my profession and my business was not serving the life that I wanted to live. I had been working with multiple mentors and coaches over the years and one particular coach in 2012 assisted me with my realizations that I needed a radical change in my life.

Just at that time, I was contacted by a teammate I played rugby with, who is in Thailand. They needed a couple of doctors to come work there with them. I thought to myself, "All I need to work are my hands. My hands are my business." So I packed everything up and ended up spending more than a year and a half in Thailand.

Many magical and life-changing things happened to me there. I was touched by the kindness and openness of people in south east Asia, like the tuk-tuk driver who showed me around and welcomed me into his family during an unexpected week long stay to reinstate my Visa. This led to me doing a clinical outreach trip where I witnessed many miracles. I had a lineup of people wanting me to lay my hands on them. It was an absolute honor, humbling and mind expanding at the same time. That moment in my life has shaped my professional career profoundly.

My second low point was an even deeper type of pain

than the first one, however the redirection led to even deeper fulfillment in my life.

Sharpening the Saw

"The 7 Habits of Highly Effective People" by Stephen Covey has been a huge influence in my life. "Sharpen the saw" is his seventh habit, in essence means to take the time to refine and improve your skills. This has been the theme in my life and practice since I came back to the US in 2015.

I'm in the relationship I have always wanted, with my partner Giuliana, and we have a beautiful daughter who delights and challenges me daily. My practice and business is set up in a way that lights me up and allows me to serve my patients' "highest good". All of these blessings have been the result of my two all time lows.

To me, sharpening the saw means daily practices and continually listening to the guidance I receive from events, my body and intuition and using the lessons I receive to build my visions and desires. I know that I am on the right track because it feels so good and things just keep working out for me. I also accept there may be a next low point, if that is what it takes to bump me up to the next level.

Serving my patients also helps me sharpen the saw. As I help people overcome their pain and struggles, I learn just as much, if not more, than they do. Whether they have fairly straight forward complaints or very complex cases that no other practitioner has been able to solve, I know that the pain and the problems in their lives are the result of them living out of alignment with who they really are. As I help them to overcome the pain, they get a better life as a side effect.

My Awareness, Awakening and Healing System

Professional training, clinical experience and lessons learned from the low points in my life have helped me to devise the Awareness, Awakening and Healing System that I use in my practice. The steps are the same whether I work with someone who thinks that their condition is too far gone to help or a person who has a new symptom or condition that is disrupting their life. The results never cease to amaze me and it is always a privilege and honor to get to support someone with my work.

Many of the people who come to me are having a health crisis. They are in pain and are dissatisfied with their health and well-being. They commonly feel like:

- This is not who I am
- This is not the path I want to be on
- I'm on a runaway train
- I'm going downhill too fast
- Can I turn this around before it's too late?
- How did I get here?
- I can't take this anymore
- This has to change

No matter how long term, chronic or difficult the problem is or whether you have tried everything and nothing has worked, it is possible to live a happy, healthy and pain-free life. You can move from feeling trapped, in pain and out-of-control, to feeling great and empowered in every aspect of your life by restoring proper balance and function to the body, mind and soul.

I do this by working with my patients through five simple steps.

1. **Crisis Control.** This step is like triage. We want to relieve the pain and take immediate action to stop the bleeding, so to speak. We make the abrupt change that is needed.

2. **Get the Wake up Call.** Once we wake up, we need to see what track we're on. If this track does not take us where we want to go, we need to decide which track to switch to, in order to get where we want.

3. **Stop Feeding the Fire.** We remove all habits, thoughts and behaviors that support the problem we're experiencing. When we're barreling along down the wrong track, we need to slow the momentum down before we can change tracks.

4. **Build Momentum Towards the Life You Want.** We consistently take small incremental action steps to support our life short-term and long term goals. We create a picture of where we want to be in a year and at age 80, 90 or beyond.

5. **Sharpen the Saw.** We continually review and adjust our habits, thoughts and behaviors so that we get better and better, age gracefully and maximize life's enjoyment.

By looking at a patient's health through the perspective of their whole life, this system has allowed me to get phenomenal breakthroughs with people with all sorts of conditions, from very diverse backgrounds and varying degrees of hope and belief.

When Lydia came in to see me she was 55 years old. She had two knee replacements, could hardly walk and felt like an old lady. She was married to a very active Vietnam vet and their favorite thing to do together was walking on the beach. She was severely overweight, waddled to get around and felt like her life was over.

We worked together for six months through the steps of my Awareness, Awakening and Healing System and got dramatic results. She continued to apply the strategies and tools she learned on her own. When I ran into her another six-months later, I hardly recognized her. She had been walking on the beach with her husband and because of the mindset shifts she achieved from my system, she had lost over 100 pounds. She now seems younger and feels better at 60 then she did when she was 55 years old.

When Doug came into my office, he was a tough, grumpy, hard-working 60-year-old electrician. He smokes, bowls and doesn't believe anything he can't see with his own eyes. The only reason he came to see me was that he ran out of options and he wasn't afraid to tell me that. He was a total mess. He had restless leg syndrome, sciatica, back pain, tremors in his left arm, his knees were shot and he had high pressure in his eyes. He was actually considering building a wheelchair ramp on his house because he anticipated not being able to walk in the near future. He was still dealing with the effects of a very messy divorce and feared for his livelihood.

After his first session with me, he stood up and said," you are a god". His arm stopped shaking and his back and leg pain were gone. After working through my Awareness,

Awakening and Healing System for the next year, his legs were no longer restless, his knees were almost 100% and he was eating better and taking supplements that work. A bonus side effect that I found out about later was that he no longer had erectile dysfunction. This had very positive effects in his new relationship which has since progressed to marriage.

Doug and his new wife Susan now come to see me together for their treatment. He no longer internalizes his feelings and their relationship continues to deepen. He also informed me that he gets regular compliments on how good his posture is for his age.

While my work is great for people with old, chronic conditions and situations that may seem too far gone to help, it also works wonders with the very young. One of my favorite success stories ever, is that of a little boy named Matthew. His mom brought him in when he was four years old on a recommendation from one of her friends. They had been to see every specialist in the Tri-State area because he was going blind.

We began working through my Awareness, Awakening and Healing System and I focused on a severe nerve distortion in his upper neck. Within a month his mom noticed he was holding books further away from his face and that he was getting more confident and athletic. After three months, Matthew was smiling, running and playing. His eyesight continued to improve. His mom was so relieved and grateful to see her son behaving like a normal child.

He went from an intimidated little boy, to a confident athlete who is not afraid to jump into a soccer game with the other kids. While his visual acuity is not 100%, he has been able to live the life of an active child, making the best of the eyesight he does have.

What You Will Discover in this Book

If you have stuck with me so far, you are either at a turning point in your life and situations or circumstances are urging you to do something now, or you're ready to take life to a new level and you are seeking the guidance to get there. Whether life has gotten too uncomfortable for you not to change or things are too comfortable and you crave something new and exciting, you will find answers in this book. Together we'll be busting some myths, exploring new vantage points and uncovering new meanings to events that have shaped our health and lives.

In Chapter 1, you'll discover a new and liberating way to use symptoms in your body to get the health and well-being you desire. You will begin to understand the symbolism and relationships of your life events, health conditions and desires in Chapter 2. By the end of Chapter 3 you will see that having your intentions and the right use of your energy aligned is a powerful way to manifest what you want with your health and in your life.

Chapters 4 and 5 discuss concepts and perspectives that will have you seeing everything about yourself and the way you live your life in a new light. You will explore how your body is more energy than solid and why patterns repeat themselves with your health, life events and relationships. In Chapter 6 I talk about how we can all make our lives and healing way easier by stop being our own worst enemy. Then in Chapter 7 we cover how to turbo charge your healing by upgrading your beliefs about how you heal.

In Chapters 8 and 9 I share how my patients become very empowered in all aspects of their lives and develop a deep sense of peace. This is something I want for each and every one of you and it is totally available to you no matter what state you are in. This comes when you change the story about your life and realize that everything about your life today, good or bad, is just perfect. With that, I send you on your way to make decisions and take action from that point of perfection and create the life of your visions.

Is It Time for You to Start Listening to Your Body and Living the Life You Really Want?

No matter what your age or the condition that is bothering you, you can move from feeling trapped, in pain and out-of-control, to feeling great and empowered in every aspect of your life. I love assisting people in gaining the wisdom from their body and taking action towards living life on their terms. If you want to know if I can help your situation, please contact me at contact@drkeving.com or visit DrKevinG.com. I would love to have the chance to meet you and to give you a free consultation so we can discuss the best course of action for you to restore proper balance and function to your body, mind and emotions.

It's never too late and there is always hope. I believe in miracles and have the great honor of witnessing them every day. I would love to participate in yours.

With gratitude,

Dr. Kevin

Chapter 1

Symptoms Are the Story

We all get sensations in our body from time to time, some of them positive and some of them painful, some of them annoying, and some of them downright disconcerting. These little signals that we get are called symptoms. Symptoms are the number one reason that people seek the help and advice from any type of health practitioner and they are the number one reason that people come into my office to see me.

These symptoms can represent any type of problem, for example illness in the body or problems with a particular organ like your intestines or heart. They can tell us that there is inflammation in a joint or that something is out of alignment. They alert us when we are overdoing it and they get our attention so that we do something about it. Ultimately, they cause us to change our course, our actions, and possibly the shape of our lives.

The Physical Location of Symptoms in the Body

Often times, physical symptoms are located at particular

points in the body, possibly a certain body part, joint or in a particular organ. Most people's common instinct is to come to the conclusion that the area of the symptom is the place in the body that needs to be treated. What I'd like you to explore and the discussion of this chapter is, that there are many connections to our symptoms. When we follow these connections and respond to the guidance we receive, we can find the true source of the problem and take the appropriate action to get rid of the symptom once and for all.

There are three things that we will look at in this chapter:

1. Connecting the dots on a physical level

2. The mind body connection

3. The physical/emotional relationship of symptoms

Connecting the Dots on a Physical Level

When we have pain in a particular area of our body, it is logical to assume that we should look at that body part as the source of the pain. However, we must also consider the fact that our entire body is physically connected. Remember the song from grade school, "The hip bone's connected to the leg bone, leg bone connected to the knee bone..." etc etc? All parts of the body are related to one another, whether they are side-by-side or some distance apart. When we consider these connections, we are much more likely to find the source of the problem that will get rid of the symptom permanently.

I often get my patients to place their fingers on the hip

bone also known as the greater trochanter, the big bump on the side of the upper leg, so they can feel the movement in it when they wiggle their toes. This is to show them that movement or lack of movement in one part of the body has an impact on many other parts of the body, even if they are not in close proximity.

If someone has ankle pain, the problem can originate in the foot or at some point below the level of the ankle. It could also be coming from the knee or some level above the joint. When we consider the relationship of the movement between different body parts, we can much more accurately diagnose and treat the cause of the symptoms.

For example, when I first started in practice, I had a longtime patient who stubbed her toe so badly that she had to go to the emergency room and get it immobilized with a boot. Shortly after, she had the worst case of dizziness in her life. She went back to emergency and got medications which helped her for about an hour. The dizziness persisted but it would go away whenever she came in to see me for an adjustment. Chiropractic and medication helped to address the symptoms, but did not address the cause.

The day she took the boot off was the date dizziness stopped for good. It had added a half inch to her height on one side and internally this created a tilt to her head to compensate and keep her eyes level. This lady was over 70 and this imbalance pressured a nerve in her upper neck that caused the dizziness. This just goes to show you that a problem at the level of your foot, or your little toe to be more specific, can create symptoms as far away as your head.

The Mind Body Connection

Not only are physical parts of the body connected, but the mind and body are also linked. In particular, the brain is connected to every part of the body through a network of nerves. The level of nerve connection between the brain and body dictates how much and how precise the control of that area can be. For example, the hands require a great deal of direction for the complex movements that they perform. However, the elbow do not require the same amount of complexity in its control. What we see, is that the number of neurons to the hand far exceed number of neurons to elbow.

In fact, if we draw a representation of the body that is proportionate in size to the number of neurons that supply it, we get a very funny looking picture. Some parts of the body that are very small but require fine motor control appear very big in this picture, whereas other parts that are quite large but don't require as much control, appear very small. This picture is called a motor homunculus, as shown below.

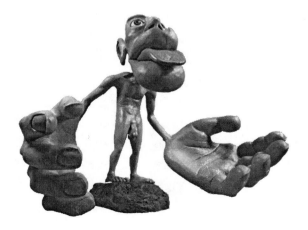

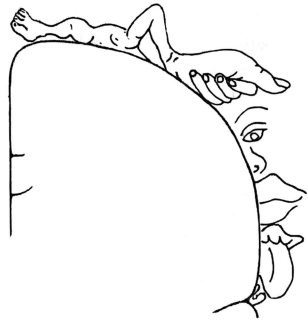

Since all parts of the body are connected to the brain via neurons, it makes sense that our thoughts control the movement and function of our body. We never actually think specifically that we want to move our hand. We just do it. But lots of activity goes on in your head in order to get your hand to produce the very skilled behaviors that we are used to everyday. We often take for granted how much communication is happening between the brain and the rest of the body, in order for us to enjoy the ease of the simplest of tasks. How then, do you think repeated thoughts that you have about yourself, your body, or how you relate to the world around you, affect the function of your body?

For example, one of my patients was a woman with sacral pain, that is a pain in her lower back and buttocks.

I had seen her many times before and chiropractic adjustments got temporary relief of her pain. But the pain kept coming back and she wanted to find the source of it.

While I was doing an assessment with her, she revealed that she was having hard time with her mom. She said that, "Her mom is being a real pain in the butt". When I asked her about what she meant, she said, "All women that have kids are a pain in the butt". I then stated, "You have children, correct?" "Yes" was her answer. I then said, "and who has a pain in the butt?" Of course she said that she did and we laughed at the whole thing. But then this.

This thought pattern cued me to look for a blockage pattern of the cranium, because I suspected that her buttock pain had a mental component. Her thought pattern had become a self fulfilling prophecy. She suddenly realized that she was a woman with children and that she had manifested pain in her butt. Releasing the physical blockage associated at the cranium and add her awareness of the limiting thought pattern, took care of the low back and buttock pain for good. Now whenever she gets pain, she looks at her life and connects the dots herself.

But it's not just what we think about that affects our body. How we feel emotionally can also cause changes in our body, that lead to symptoms.

The Physical/Emotional Relationship of Symptoms

We all know that when we are in a bad mood, things appear worse and when we are in good mood they appear better. We get sick when we're under stress and pain feels more intense when we are upset. Our emotional state has a very big impact on our body and how it feels.

In the brain, the physical component of our brains' motor nervous system is directly next to the emotional and sensory parts of the brain. There are lots of neutral networks intertwined between the mental, physical and emotional components of our existence.

The most obvious connection between how we feel emotionally and the physical state of our body is body language. We are all experts at reading posture to understand other people's emotional state.

Think about it. If you see somebody moving along slowly, with slouched shoulders and their head down, you will likely assume that they are sad, they've had a hard day or they are depressed. Conversely, if you see someone moving briskly with the shoulders back and whistling, smile on their face, you will probably think they are in a great mood or that they got good news.

People recognize a lot about someone's mental and emotional state from their body language. In fact some experts say that body language is responsible for as much as 70 to 90% of communication.

The reason for this is that emotions in humans are experienced physically through the way we move, breath and speak. My four month old daughter responds to my facial expressions and the tone of my voice. It's inherently built in. Picking up on the Emotional State of others is an inborn mechanism that has allowed humans to not only survive but to thrive.

For this reason, whenever I am examining a patient

for a physical problem, I'm always listening for cues about their thoughts and emotions that are likely contributing to the symptoms they are experiencing. To me, symptoms are just the outcome of the stories that someone has about the way they are experiencing life and how easy or hard they perceive it to be.

You can spend a lifetime with a practitioner, doctor, therapist or any other helpful person, chasing symptoms and relieving them, be it with spinal adjustments, medications, supplements, herbs or exercise. This is the reason that many people have chronic problems that will not go away. This is also why I have had such a great success in helping people heal from problems where no one else could help.

Whenever people heal, it is because they have moved beyond the symptoms and explored their story. This is actually the purpose of symptoms. Symptoms have a symbolic meaning and they're to guide us to investigate something. They relate to a story that we are holding onto about who we are, who we are not, or what we are doubting or fulfilling about ourselves.

If you really want to get to the bottom of your symptoms, take a good look at your life. Everything in life is symbolic and your body reflects how you feel about what is going on. In the next chapter we will discuss life's symbolism and how you can use it to find your path to vibrant health.

Chapter 2

Life Is Symbolic

Many people are searching for the meaning of life and would love it if someone would just tell them something that could make sense of everything that's happening around them. Wouldn't it be nice if there was an answer that could tell you what it's all about, why you are here and what this crazy thing that just happened means?

What if life had no meaning other than what you decided it was all about? What if this life is all about you, your thoughts, your desires and whether you are living authentically on your terms? If we start here, life can become really fun, much easier and an amazing masterpiece that we are guided to create.

Life is symbolic, meaning that we are always getting signs about how we are living, how we are perceiving the events around us and the action we are taking in response to them. When we don't pay attention to what's going on around us, it can seem like life is a series of random events that just happen to us. When you are constantly in a reactive mode, things stress you out and you don't understand why this is happening to you.

But life is always giving you signs and telling you whether you are on track with your reason for being here or if you should be taking a different path to get what you want.

What Is a Symbol?

A symbol can be defined as an object that has meaning. For example a get well card can be symbolic of the caring that you are expressing for someone. A diamond ring is a symbol of commitment, love and security. When someone is proposing marriage, the diamond ring represents the commitment and love in the relationship.

Symbolism can be found in all sorts of objects and occurrences in our lives. We are simply relating an external object or event to a feeling, thought or perspective that we have inside.

When I made a decision to sell my practice and move to Thailand, things in my life began to move very quickly. I had a very short time to tie up all the loose ends, get my life in order and leave the country. I had to sit down and have a conversation with my family and write a letter to my patients, not to mention all the other obligations that needing tending to before leaving the country.

I started getting really bad right shoulder and neck pain. I went to my chiropractor and I saw someone to get energy work done on me. While this alleviated some of the pain, the symptom would not go away. In fact, my neck and shoulder did not stop hurting until a few days after I landed in Thailand.

Now why would I be getting this neck and right shoulder pain? If I considered the symbolism in my life, I was feeling stressed by the opinions and perceptions of others. I was going about sharing the message of my leaving the same way I had always gone about things. My standard approach to handling these issues took into account my needs but perhaps was a bit inconsiderate of the other people and commitments in my life.

Pain in the shoulder is often representative of taking on responsibility. The throat and neck are commonly related to communication and talking. Knowing this, I took steps to become more confident and really okay with making the move. But the pain did not go away.

As the move date was nearing, I worked two straight days getting packed and was running around doing last-minute errands. I was still dealing with the responsibility of what people thought of my actions and I had a fear of how they would judge me.

As I went through the experience, most were excited for me and very supportive, even though some did not agree. At the end of the day, they all wanted what was best for me. I came to the conclusion that everything was working out for me. I wonder what would have happened if I had come to that realization in the first place. Would I have had to suffer through those symptoms?

Once I arrived in Thailand and got over the time difference, I had this complete relaxing in my mind that I did make the right move and I had to do this for me in my life. I knew that it was okay and the sense of responsibility for what people thought of me and my actions went away and so did the pain.

Recognizing the symbolism in your life comes down

to your self-awareness for how you feel living your life on your own terms versus the importance of the thoughts and opinions of others. There is sort of personal sovereignty that is necessary. As they say on the airplane, put your oxygen mask on first before assisting another person.

The Importance of Selfishness

It is very important to realize and develop the value of your self. When you have a high self worth, you'll have a much easier time taking action on your wants and desires. You will be much less concerned about what others think. This is a very difficult concept for many of us because we have learned a very negative definition of selfishness.

From the negative perspective, being selfish means putting yourself above others without any regard for anyone else. We relate this to ruthless people with a mentality of achieving their goals by doing whatever it takes, disregarding the consequences of their actions and hurting others in the long run. They will undercut others, lie and cheat. In this perspective all the energy is one directional. There is no flow back-and-forth and it all flows towards yourself.

Because of this negative perspective on selfishness, most people have an aversion towards focusing on the self. It is something they have learned is right and good to do. They don't consider the positive side of selfishness, which can involve doing things to rejuvenate and regenerate yourself, so that you can be better for others. If you are so focused on giving to others but don't take care of yourself, you have nothing to give. There is a balance between rejuvenating and giving and to caring for yourself and caring for others.

This is a rampant problem for mothers who are trying to be the new superwoman. They are burning the candle at both ends and taking a lighter to the middle. This leads to a variety of health problems, including adrenal fatigue and burnout. Many people turn to coffee, alcohol and drugs or binge eating in the middle of the night to stuff down emotions. They are stressed out with no time for themselves.

Symbols in our lives can show us where our behaviors are out of whack with our desires, how we need to grow and change, and when something is not serving us anymore. Symbols may yield the inspiration for an idea, the solution to a problem or the final key you have been searching for to get you to the next step.

Use Your Awareness to Find the Symbols in Your Life

Awareness is a very interesting thing that can determine how we take in what's going on in our environment. Awareness is the perception of what is going on inside you and around you. There are many levels and it is a matter of using your mind and senses to take notice and assign and be aware of meaning.

Some examples of the expanding awareness include learning a new word or getting a new car. Your friend may introduce you to a new word that you have never heard of before. Once you learned how to say, spell and define the word, you start to see it everywhere and you hear it used in conversation frequently, and this seemingly occurs suddenly. Maybe you are about to get a new car, you have picked out the make, model and color and you're very excited. All of a sudden you start seeing this car that you have never noticed before everywhere on the roads. Awareness works this way. Whatever you notice, you seem to get more of.

There is a part of the brain called the reticular activating system, that is in charge of things like this. When you put an idea in the mind, the mind seeks it out and you start seeing it. Before you focus on it, your brain does not place importance and it informs you to ignore it. Once there is a desire to know more about it, you cross the threshold and its appearance stands out and truth is revealed, it feels odd.

These are external examples but we can also consider how awareness works within us. People can notice aches and pains within the body. These can be quite blatant, like throbbing headaches, stabbing low back pain or tingling in the arm. They can also be quite subtle, like thoughts, feelings or a gut instinct. Some people act on this gut instinct while other people ignore it. With awareness, we can start to see a level of connection inside our bodies and outside, in our lives.

Often times, people do not notice the symbols and signs that they get inside their body until they are blatant. They are unaware of the subtle cues their body is giving them, to alert them to discrepancies between what they are doing and what they really want in their lives. There can be a lot of noise from other thoughts in our head that seem more urgent and demand attention right away.

Back to my Thailand story, it was getting down to the wire, I was leaving in just three weeks, and things just needed to get done. The way I was communicating with people was not in alignment with who I was and how much

I cared for them. I needed to shift my communication with my family, friends and my patients. I ignored the need to quiet my body.

If I had taken some time to allow the stillness I had needed so I could focus on the more subtle feelings in my body, I would have noticed the signs that were telling me to address the situation in a better, smoother way. My body was talking to me and telling me I was going to do something that was not the greatest good for my family and my life. I was repeating the same old pattern, the same way I dealt with problems and feelings in the past, that had made me very sick.

I did eventually get the message, and the symptoms did alleviate, once I landed in Thailand. I could have handled the situation so much more elegantly with the guidance of the subtle symbols in my body and life. The reason that I did not was because I was not aware of the internal and external symbols. I was learning.

Inside out or Outside in

The symbolism in life can work in either direction. You can have symbols inside your body, often known as symptoms, telling you about the meaning you are assigning to situations in your life's environment. You can also have symbols outside in your environment cueing you to feelings inside your body.

My story about neck and shoulder pain is an example of the symbols on the inside that reflect my reaction to external circumstances. How then do we get external symbols that reflect what's going on inside us?

In shamanic healing, the study of ancient cultures' health and medicinal practices, we often encounter animal totems that show up to give us signs. Early on when I was discovering my healing modalities beyond chiropractic care, I had many experiences with interesting things happening in my life. I would have strange interactions with animals. These would involve almost hitting cats, dogs, or snakes with my car or something like a butterfly landing in my hand or a deer locking eyes with me. The animal in question would represent how I was dealing with something in my life.

Just before I left for Thailand, I was covering the practice of a friend, who ran a very structural and biomechanical chiropractic practice. At the time I had some internal conflict with practicing this way because I was much more holistic and seeking the energetic/emotional components of health.

One evening, when I got home to my parents house just before covering for my friend, there was a raccoon waiting for me in the driveway. In all the years that we have been in that house, I had never seen a raccoon there before. It just sat there in the driveway staring at me. It finally left and I went into the house to look up the meaning. Raccoons have the symbolism of wearing a mask. When I read more about it, I found that it was okay to sometimes be a different person in cases where you needed to help someone else. Even though I felt that I had moved beyond this style of practice, I could still be of great service to those patients. I have the skills and did not need to feel that I was being a fraud.

One of my patients kept getting the symbol of a peacock appearing to her. They would show up in her dreams and in pictures, so we looked up the meaning of the peacock. The peacock has to do with expressing your full colors. She realized that she had not been expressing herself fully. This woman had become more beautiful as she matured in life, however she covered herself up and kept her greatest attributes hidden within. She did not think she had anything to show.

She shifted her thinking and started to be more bold. She embraced an exotic component within herself and began putting herself out there, living more gracefully. Now she is buying new clothes, getting dressed up and going out, spending time with friends and meeting men. She is enjoying the new chapter of her life and the expression of everything she has become.

How to Start Seeing the Symbolism in Your Life

There are always symbols that are guiding us towards the life of our visions. When you have guidance like this, it is a shame to not be taking it. You can start to notice and respond to symbols in your life and use them to shape your future.

Has something been showing up in your life multiple times a week? What is it trying to tell you? In my office I often hear patients saying to me "Doc! That's the third time I've heard that this week." I always ask them, "What is that saying to you?"

Trying to understand what symbols mean for you in

your life is a discovery process. You must ask yourself how this applies in your life and what you need to take action on. If a pain suddenly comes on within you, ask yourself what you were just thinking about. Compare this thought to location of the pain. For example the hands represent something we are holding onto. The feet often indicate action steps are necessary. Shoulders have to do with responsibility, as we saw in my story about moving to Thailand. What does the body part have to do with what you were just thinking?

In **Appendix 1: Body Parts, Associated Emotions and Possible Symbolism**, I have compiled a chart from traditional Chinese medicine, applied kinesiology and energy medicine. Although the meaning of your symptoms may not be this cut and dry, it is definitely a starting point for finding the meaning and receiving guidance.

Once we start to gain insights into the symbols in our lives, we begin to see that they are strongly connected to our intentions and guiding us with morality. This is the guidance you receive when you are authentically aligned with who you are and what you want in life. When you listen to it, things go smoothly. When you are out of alignment, it can get rough and there maybe some symbols that are there to guide you back to the path.

It is up to us to be aware of these symbols and take the right action steps to get our lives back on track. When I was preparing for my move to Thailand, my intention was to get things done, no matter what came my way. I was using selfishness the wrong way and did not go about things in the best way. By not considering the actions and consequences,

I was not using my intention and all the energies involved in the best possible way. This is the concept of right use-ness, which we will discuss in the next chapter. Simply put, right use-ness is combining action, intent and energy in a way to achieve the best possible outcome for all involved.

The woman with the peacock totem was an intelligent person and her intention was to get out there, have more fun and experience more grace. She chose a positive path of changing her hair, buying new clothes and planning more outings. This right use-ness supported her growth and happiness. Had she not taken these actions, she would have continued down the path of depression

Chapter 3

Intention and Right Use-ness

In Chapter 2, we talked about symbolism and the relationship between symptoms in your body, your thoughts and feelings about life. Understanding that there's a connection and applying this idea can help you resolve pain once and for all. When it becomes clear to you that pain is simply an indication that something needs to change, you can take action and get back on course with what you want in your body and your life.

As I help my patients heal the root cause of their pain and they begin to understand how to use their body signals to guide their decisions and perception of their circumstances, they begin to see how much control they have over their life and health. They begin to see a new usefulness to pain and symptoms, as they are guided to heal not only their body but their emotions and their lives as well.

We begin to see that life will always have pain but that we need not fear it. It is useful and beneficial in assisting us to live our best life on the physical, mental and spiritual level. This does not need to make sense right away, however, it just starts to become clear as the symptoms drop away and patients begin to enjoy movement and function in their bodies, free of pain.

When my patients heal from and resolve issues completely, it becomes important for them to live in a way that will make sure that they never experience the undesired problem or disease again. Our work together helps them develop their own power over the health of their bodies and their lives. They work with me on a new level, where I guide them to influence their thoughts and emotions in a way that gets the ease and flow of movement in their body to match the ease of flow in their life experience.

The concepts of intention and right use-ness become very important at this stage. Intention is defined as an aim or a plan, a design or an outcome. Right use-ness is a term that I will describe in more detail later. For now, think of an intention as the goal and right use-ness as the way we go about getting there.

One of my mentors, Dr. James Chestnut, uses the picture frame principle to describe intention. You want to frame the result you wish to achieve and create a picture that you can see. You want to know what it looks like in the short, medium and long term.

When people have intention, they stop just letting life happen to them and begin to focus on their desire for a particular outcome. Intention is a purpose. It has yet to occur or is about to occur. The majority of people live without any intention other than avoidance of things they do not like or immediate gratification from a particular action or event. But there are so many ways that intention can be used to experience much more joy and ease in every moment of our lives.

As they heal from their immediate pains, my patients learn to do so through intention. They take responsibility for how they are observing the sensations in their body and decide to experience them from a new emotional level.

Intention sets the tone for what is being discussed. Setting the tone is a decision about the emotion we want to feel as we move through a set of circumstances. In my practice, when someone has back pain, the intention is to be fully comfortable in walking, standing and sleeping. They want to have free mobility. The general tone or background, as we get closer to accomplishing the goal of being pain free, becomes very important. The general tone is that we want to feel good. The specificity is in visualizing, actually imagine seeing yourself standing in the grocery line, driving a car or picking up your child and having a pleasant experience performing these activities with emotions that demonstrate you are feeling good.

Setting the intention for a particular goal or outcome is only part of the puzzle. The next piece is how we plan to use our energy and efforts to achieve the particular result we seek. There are many ways we can go about directing our energy to create a particular end. The end justifies the means, but we are responsible for our choice of the path we choose to get there. I call this concept right use-ness.

The term right use-ness was coined by a mentor of mine, named Carol Gold. She is a retired lawyer, life coach, radio personality and my spiritual guru. I define right use-ness as the way we use our actions and energy to achieve the intention that we desire.

Right use-ness is a concept that we apply to our lives

with awareness. There is a lot of self-analysis associated
with applying right use-ness in our lives. It is a practice of
daily awareness that involves perceiving how one interacts
with themselves and others. It is very personal and experienced differently by everyone who applies it. Yet it is something that must be applied in order to experience the benefit or experience the consequences of breaking natural law.

One learns to apply the concept of right use-ness by observing the outcomes they have achieved in their lives and
analyzing their effects on others and whether they would
choose to use the path that got them there again or if there
is a more efficient, respectful, honorable, satisfying path.

There are three components to the practice of right
use-ness. These are:

1. The thoughts and motives we have about our in-
    tention

2. The feelings or emotions we experience regarding
    this intention

3. The actions we take in attempts to realize this in-
    tention

For someone who is in pain and unable to walk prop-
erly, their desire maybe to walk better at work and at home.
A natural way to achieve this could be to use chiropractic alignments but there are also other choices. They may
choose to go the pharmaceutical route and numb the pain
with drugs. In more serious cases they may go with a surgical intervention. The question is, what is the best decision
for the body in the long-term?

In business we may want to create a certain level of

financial gain and there are many ways to achieve this. There are honest and ethical means, that take into consideration the highest good of everyone involved. There are also illegal, immoral and backstabbing approaches. We may be able to arrive at the same outcome of acquiring a certain amount of money but our choice of path can have dramatic implications on our long-term happiness and fulfillment.

What happens when you start applying the practice of right use-ness?

1. You find yourself at peace with your interactions and decisions daily

2. Internal struggle drops away because your intentions create ease when making decisions

3. Interactions become easy and you maintain bridges instead of burning them

4. You get a sense in your life that you're building something great

5. You create a sense of self, based around the upbeat and positive way you go about things

Difficult interactions that people usually avoid such as ending a relationship can occur in a gratifying and mutually beneficial way. Because most people avoid situations that they do not enjoy, the end result is achieved in a way that negatively impacts everyone. You may find situations like somebody cheating, name-calling, or being cruel that forces the other person to leave. The positive way to achieve this could be a cordial conversation or letter, without blame or the need to put the other person down. With the goal of explaining that this relationship is not working in the best way for the highest good of both people, it can be obvious that the best choice is to move on to greener pastures.

Here is how to consider the three components of right use-ness in the example above:

Thought-avoid and hurt versus take responsibility and consider what is the greatest good of all involved;

Emotion-avoidance, resentment and malice versus consideration, respect and honesty;

Action-underhanded, self-gratification versus open communication and agreement.

When working with the concepts of intention and right use-ness, the most important thing to understand, is that the feeling you have in everything you do, affects you, your body and those around you.

Candace Pert, author of the book *Molecules of Emotion*, showed that the thoughts and emotions we experience affect the production of neurotransmitters that change the receptivity of our nerve tissues. Negative emotions can in fact make our nerve endings more sensitive to pain, while positive emotions can cause our nerves to stimulate more pleasant feelings.

Professor Imoto, from Japan, performed experiments where he observed the crystallization pattern of water that had been placed in the field of different emotions. The results were dramatic and consistently showed that when you froze water that was exposed to positive emotions, you got a beautiful and orderly crystallization pattern. Water that had been subjected to the field of negative emotions crystallized in disorderly, harsh patterns. With our bodies being such a high percentage of water and perpetually existing in the field of our emotions, our decision to keep our emotions positive is of the utmost importance.

When I was practicing in Thailand I had the opportunity to work with a British woman for 3 to 4 months. She had terrible health problems that were extremely disruptive to her life. She had debilitating headaches, jaw pain and her right leg was swollen and next to useless. She wanted freedom from her pain and disease. We established that her intention was to be more comfortable and steady in her body.

It was obvious to me that there was major emotional discord that accompanied all of the dysfunction in her body. She soon revealed that she had major emotional problems with every member of her family. Her biggest issue was the relationship with her son, whom she had not spoken to in several years. It seemed to her as though the family that he had married into, did not get along with her family and that he had chosen his new family over her. She had a deep desire to reconnect with him but every time she sent him an email or letter she got no response.

In treating her pain, I worked with the concept of intention and right use-ness. I had her start to visualize what it would feel like if her son reached out and called her. She told me that it would be an exciting breakthrough. When I asked her what that experience would feel like, she had no idea. So I asked her to describe the feeling with terms like hard or soft, bubbly or rough and round or square. I wanted her to have a sense of the feeling of the word she used and how the experience of the emotion would feel in her body.

When she thought of her son, she started to create a warm, bubbly and expansive feeling that she associated with an exciting breakthrough. I would guide her into that feeling every time she came in for a treatment. Because her body had been under the influence of negative emotions for so long, there were areas of tension and resistance that were unable to respond to the warm, bubbly, expansive feeling. My clinical judgment guided me to those areas of her body, where I would perform chiropractic adjustments, reiki or other such modalities.

Every time I performed a treatment with her, I held the vision of what she would look and feel like in the experience of reconnecting with her son. I would see her walking into my office with a big smile on her face and telling me all about the conversation she had with him as though it had already happened.

She had been coming in to see me once a week. The week after a wonderful release during an adjustment, which eased her body's resistance to experiencing an exciting breakthrough, she came in overflowing with excitement and telling me her son had contacted her on Facebook and that they had set up a time to do a video call. All her symptoms dramatically improved. But just as there was still work to be done in the relationship with her son, there was much work to be done to help her body heal.

Over the next few weeks we continued to work on her perception of the relationship with her son. She saw dramatic healing and began to experience much more joy as she allowed herself to be accepted into his family. I only got to work with her for another three months, in which time her pain became manageable and she was able to walk. Had I been able to spend the time necessary to help her heal all the relationships in her family, my prognosis is that she would have returned her body to a 100 percent state of health.

The British patient wasn't focused on what she wanted and in her frustration was blaming everyone to their face. She was yelling and getting into arguments and she built tension within and between people. This led to her being cut out of the family. By trying to be right all the time and not accepting her responsibility in the situation, she had put her energy to the wrong use for achieving her desire of acceptance. When her intention of healing the relationship with her son and being accepted into the family became clear, she understood that this use of her energy had been the cause of major pain in her body and life. By applying right use-ness of her energy, she was able to experience intense healing in all aspects of herself.

To apply the three components of right use-ness:

Thought-negative, confrontational, not taking responsibility versus accepting, seeing her role, and forgiving;

Feeling-resentment, anger and sadness versus exciting and expansive emotions that she wanted to feel;

Action-blame, self absorption and self-pity versus developing a daily practice and feeling her desired outcome accompanied with chiropractic adjustments.

The circumstances that we encounter in life are always going to cause disruption to the way that we are are used to living. This can cause pain in the short term, however, it presents an opportunity for us to shape our life into exactly what we want. Problems tell you when you are off-track and they have the amazing ability to knock us back onto track towards what we want.

When we live with intention and we practice right use-ness we are able to take an active role in creating life on our terms. We stop being victims of circumstance and we start being creators of our destiny.

Chapter 4

You are Energy

In the last chapter we talked about how the right use of your focus and energy has a huge impact on how your body heals. The focus that you maintain around the situations and circumstances in your life is always affecting the state of your body. In this chapter, we will cover why your body is so susceptible to the energy of your thoughts and emotions.

So let's consider this wonderful body of ours and how it is all held together. If you think back to science class and your experience with a microscope, no matter how in-depth you got, you know that there is a lot more to your body that you don't see. When we zoom in, we start seeing what the body is made up of.

We can see that the different areas of the body have different organs and that all of the organs are made of different types of tissues which are composed of individual cells with various rolls. As we zoom in more, we see that the cells have parts, like the nucleus and the mitochondria, if your memory of biology class serves you well.

We could continue to zoom in if we had an electron microscope and see the atoms. Zooming in still further, we

would see the protons, neutrons and electrons: the little solar system-like things within the universe of our body.

The protons and neutrons are bound together in the
nucleus and have a positive charge. The electrons orbit the
nucleus and are held there because of their negative charge.
All these positive and negative charges are responsible for
these atoms sticking together and forming our cells, tissues
and organs.

To give you a perspective, if the nucleus of the atom
was the size of a tennis ball, the electrons orbiting it would
occupy the space the size of a football stadium. When you
think of it this way, this solid body that we move around in,
is actually way more empty space than it is anything solid.
All of this organization of cells and tissue is made up of the
little atoms and is all held together by these positive and
negative forces.

Now the number of cells in our body is astronomical.
There is an incredible amount of organization and intelligence that makes this clumping together of little solar systems function as us. Can you imagine what it would take to
build a walking, talking, feeling and thinking human being
out of trillions upon trillions of little atoms?

As wonderfully complex as we are, with all the elabo-
rate functions that take place inside us, it is all held together and powered by the positive and negative charges that
create structure and allow transmission of energy. Isn't it
amazing how the simplicity and elegance of these atoms
can come together and form the organization and complexity of a human?

With this perspective of our bodies, we can see how made of energy more than being of a solid makeup.

So then let's consider the impact of energy and charge on our bodies. For example, if we are wearing socks and drag our feet across the carpet in a dry environment and then touch a metal doorknob, we get a shock. This happens because we become electrically charged and that electricity wants to release and pass through us into the doorknob.

In fact our bodies respond significantly to electromagnetic fields. We see this in medicine all the time for the use of medical imaging. MRI or magnetic resonance imaging works by subjecting the body to an electromagnetic field and then capturing the energetic response of the body through an imaging process. This allows us to visualize what is happening inside the body.

We also use the electrostatic nature of the body to observe how the brain and heart are working. We can attach leads and electrodes to the area of the body near the heart and measure the electrical impulses emitted to get a sense of how the heart is functioning with an EKG or electrocardiogram. An EEG or electroencephalogram, uses leads and electrodes attached to the head to measure brain waves.

When someone is suffering from carpal tunnel syndrome, that is nerve pain in the arm, wrist and hand, we can measure how well nerve impulses are being transmitted through the ulnar nerve with a nerve conduction test. This is accomplished by sticking needles directly into the arm and using leads connected to a device that measures the flow of electrical charge.

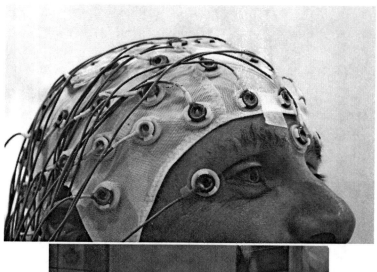

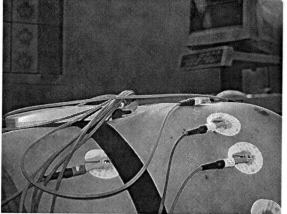

As you can see, the electrical nature of the body is very important to consider. This is why we have to be conscious about the amount of radiation, wi-fi, cell phone and other power sources we are exposed to. Medical science has invented all sorts of technologies to observe the electrical nature of the body. There's also technology available to positively impact our bodies and treat problems that occur in these energetic fields.

It becomes very important for us then, to consider the impact of anything we do that creates a variance in the energetic field of our body and what it does to our health and well-being. Unfortunately, in our western culture and medicine, there is not a lot of significance given to our energetic nature. But just because it's not addressed does not mean that it is not happening.

In eastern medicine they talk about the flow of Chi or life force. This is used in acupuncture and Qigong, to treat conditions and to increase the health of our bodies. It is used in martial arts to channel power and force, generating much more impact in a blow, than is created from simple muscular strength.

Different professions and practices have various names for this flow of energy but they're all talking about the same thing. In chiropractic, we call it innate intelligence. This is the intelligence or energy that takes half a cell from a woman and half a cell from a man and puts them together to grow a 6 foot, 200 pound human who moves, runs, thinks and creates. It is the energy that knows how to heal the body from a cut and how to fight bacteria and viruses so that we recover from illness.

When we respect this flow of innate intelligence, it takes care of us with no effort at all. When we interfere with it and create a blockage in the flow, we start to see imbalances happen in the body. Though it may have been developing for some time, our first warning that there is an imbalance comes as a signal which can take the form of pain or a sensation of dis-ease. Not feeling at ease or feeling out of sorts is the start of disease. These are the symptoms that we try so hard to treat with all sorts of medical interventions.

Symptoms however are just the messenger. They are alerting us to an imbalance in the flow of the life force. Treating the symptoms and hoping to get better is like shooting the messenger. What we need to be focusing on is the message. We want to know where the energy is blocked and how to get the innate intelligence to flow again.

"Treating the symptoms and hoping to get better is like shooting the messenger"

This is the role that I play in a person's health and healing. I connect my knowledge of the body and the energies that are associated with it, with the symptoms and life situations that my patients present with. My examination checks the different systems, how they're working and if they are functioning well or if there's a problem. I check the muscular and skeletal system, the nervous system and the acupuncture meridians to find out what is out of balance and how the body has compensated for the blockage. I check for energetic matches to toxins and pathogens as well as provide the appropriate solutions.

I want to emphasize that, when I examine a person with any condition or complaint, I never consider that there is something wrong with that person. In fact there is nothing wrong in their body. They have simply adapted to the resources that they have available. They have found the best balance possible, given the way they are dealing with their circumstances. This new balance may turn into an issue that the person may perceive as a problem but I like to teach them that it is simply the body's message that is guiding them back into balance.

The question now becomes, what is the issue? The answer really depends on the sophistication of the practitioner that the person seeks. It depends on the tools that the practitioner uses. To a carpenter with a hammer, everything is a nail. In our culture, when we are sick we go to the doctor or the MD. The reason we are sick is because there is something out of balance in our structure or with our chemistry. Perhaps there's a bacteria or pathogen out of control in our body that and we have limited or no resources within to respond with therefore making us sick.

The philosophy of disease in our culture tends to have the view that something outside of us has made us ill and something external needs to be done to get us better. It may come in the form of a pill or some sort of injection to bring us back into health. In the worst cases, when things are way out of balance, we may need to cut a part of the body away or go in and repair an organ with surgery. And sometimes this is absolutely required, but in most cases the answer is not to cut something out or to medicate the feeling away.

We need to be interested in the symptoms. We have to listen to the messenger and understand the importance of the message. Only then can we understand how things got out of balance, and how we can restore that balance. If someone has high blood pressure, just giving them pills to bring the blood pressure down, does not address why the body raised the pressure in the first place. The blood pressure reading is the messenger.

When we just address the symptoms, the relief we get is temporary. This is because the body still wants to notify us of the imbalance in flow and get us to take action to restore it. We can ignore the signals, mask them, just live with them, or we can seek to learn from them.

My role in a patient's healing is to act as a guide or a mentor so to speak, who can train them to use these messages to understand the body's wisdom. My treatment does not simply provide symptom relief, although my patients always feel better as they heal. When patients work with me, they become responsible for getting the messages that the body is sending them.

The message needs to get through. Something needs to change. Innate intelligence knows what's best for you and you have to listen. So if you miss the first message, don't worry, you will get another one. And if you plug your ears, it will just get louder. Inevitably you will get the message and make the change that's necessary. It's just a question of how severe the message needs to be before you listen. You don't have to wait until you have a heart attack before you start changing your life.

To give you an example of this, a new patient of mine came in the other night with two frozen shoulders that had been getting worse over the last four years. She could not raise her arms past her shoulders.

Obviously this was causing her major physical discomfort and inconvenience and we were looking for the physical cause. As she was telling me about all the symptoms and what had happened in the last four years, she related it to the purchase of the business franchise four years ago. It has been a time of lots of stress, pressure, responsibility and drama. On top of all that she has been going through a lawsuit.

As I completed my examination, I recapped what she had told me and used the words and language that she had used to describe the events of the last four years. Because I was listening intently and reading between the lines, I was able to capture a lot more about the situation than she was actually saying in words.

She was deeply moved and felt like she had been heard for the first time in years. This created an opening and she began to disclose some deeper emotional stuff. She told me that when she was six years old, her mother passed away from cancer. Since that time she had held on to the responsibility and burden that she felt. She said that life was always piling stuff on her. I had a visual of the waitress carrying a big tray on her shoulders and more and more stuff getting piled on top of it.

Depending on whether you are experiencing a positive or negative emotion, your body posture changes. Just think of how a depressed person stands slumped over with rounded shoulders versus a confident person standing upright, chest out and shoulders back. You cannot experience the energy of an emotion without the right shape in your body.

I had her think of the phrase she had stated about life piling stuff on her, and I tested some of the reflexes of her body to gauge their response. Think of it like the knee-jerk reaction. As long as the reaction is present I know that she is still holding on to the belief. As I performed the treatment and continue to test a reflex, I watched it diminish and eventually subside. At that point I knew the treatment was complete. When I asked her to lifter arms overhead, she was able to do so without pain.

She was amazed. I explained to her that the energy of the emotions was weighing her down like cement blocks. I asked her if it would be okay if she still had the memories of her mother but without the emotional intensity. She said she was afraid that if she let go of the memories, she would forget about her mother. That's all she had to hold onto.

We began to work with her on reframing the memory of her mother and associating emotion that had a supportive energetic impact on the body. Up until then, the emotion that she associated with her mother was one of overwhelm and hopelessness. I had her allowing new energy to come. One of appreciation. Appreciation of the memories of her mother, the time she spent with her and the experience that she got in life because of these events. I had her focus on who she had become because of this experience and how she could be thankful for things she had in her life because she had been through all of that.

I noted a peace and a calm start to fill her for the first time. When she first came into my office she was anxious, revved up and nervous. Her disposition shifted dramatically by the end of our session. She left the office excited, with a cautious optimism and amazed that she could have let this burden goes so quickly.

The Energy of Emotions

Not all emotions are created equal. Some emotions are high-energy and some emotions are low-energy. Take sadness for example. If you were being sad, would you be moving a lot or a little? Would you be breathing deeply or shallowly? Would you feel like your energy was moving or stagnant? When I ask people these questions about sadness they usually say they would be moving very little, breathing shallowly, and their energy would be stagnant.

Now consider the emotion of enthusiasm. Same questions. How much movement? How deeply are you breathing? Energy flowing or feeling stagnant? More than likely you answered that you would be moving a lot, breathing deeply, and your energy would be flowing. This happens because, in order to create the energy of emotions you need to have movement. High-level emotions that feel really good involve a lot of movement because they have a lot of energy. Low-level emotions that are draining or feel bad involve very little movement because they have very little energy.

The flow of the energy is also important. When energy moves through and around your body, it tends to energize you, make you move, and lift your spirits. Though at times when we focus within on the energy flowing, we tend to stop moving and focus. It can calm us, which is a good thing but if your energy resources get stagnant, you tend to run into lower-level emotions of boredom, apathy, sadness or depression.

Dr. Russ Rosen, a chiropractic mentor of mine, has a scale for emotions. He calls it the negative 10 to positive 10 scale. In the negative numbers, we have stress and pain, chemicals and fast food, sedentary lifestyle and stressful relationships. In the positive numbers, we feel better, we exercise, seek solutions, eat healthy and take time to practice silence and have an active social life.

When a challenging circumstance occurs how we perceive it will cause certain range of emotions to be experienced. If we experience an inconvenient situation with a negative emotion, we feel bad and we tend to experience discomfort. If we experience the same situation, yet focus on staying in a positive emotional state, we tend to feel better and more comfortable. This is why, when we have pain, we tend to forget about it when we are happy or focused on something else.

Think about a time when you received bad news. Really visualize yourself in the situation hearing about the news. What is the feeling in your body. Describe the sensations. Does it make your breath increase or decrease. Does it feel like your energy is flowing or stagnant? Do you feel more relaxed or more tense? Okay now shake yourself out and take two or three full breaths.

Now think about a time when you experienced a really great moment, like receiving a gift or a surprise, winning the game, accomplishing a goal or receiving great news. What do you feel when you visualize this experience. How does it differ from visualizing the experience of receiving bad news.

When we experience negative emotions we tend to ask questions like, "Why is this happening to me?" or "Who is responsible for this?" We tend to want to blame someone, which brings in more negativity. When we are looking for the cause outside of ourselves, it looks as though the problem happens to us. It has nothing to do with us and we need an external solution.

When we experience positive emotions, it can feel like we can accomplish anything and that in any moment, there are infinite possibilities. We may think to ourselves, "I like being here!" or "I love this feeling!" We may be in appreciation of what we do have in our lives or we may feel gratitude for something that is happening. When we are looking from within at what we do have, our body matches the feeling. It feels like everything that you want is within you now, including the answer to your question. If you have a problem, the solution appears to be within reach. Focusing on a situation with positive perspective, puts the power to heal in your hands.

My role as a practitioner is to be a coach or mentor who is facilitating a person in their growth and rebalancing. This groundbreaking and positive process, happens when the patient has an aha moment and connects the dots. They make the transition from feeling stuck, like they lack something or they don't know what to do, to feeling good, and having the ability to find the solution. They also begin to feel good in their body, have better movement and a sense of knowing that their body can heal and that everything is okay. You have all you need.

My true breakthroughs with my patients happen when they realize that they are responsible for creating and cultivating that energy. It's just like a garden that needs tending. If you don't tend to your thoughts and emotions, negative thoughts and emotions get in and grow like weeds.

If you work on your mind and emotions, you can create your own environment. It's not to say that you cannot be affected by outside influence, however, you will be more centered, certain and confident. You will have the knowing that you have the life force that will allow you to overcome challenges. It is possible to build this to the point where outside influences can hardly affect you and you can adapt to any challenge.

You will never be happy if you count on external circumstances to influence your emotional state. When you're in a positive emotional state, you create your circumstances. When you're in a negative emotional state you're in for a wild ride. Challenging circumstances will arise. This is a given. But if you're not emotionally adaptable, they will sap your energy and you will always feel like a victim.

But you can develop your awareness and notice your emotional state from a place of responsibility. When you do this it becomes possible to make a decision about how you choose to feel as you move through this challenging situation. These situations give you knowledge and experience that make you stronger and help you to be of service to others. It's on your path and it helps you become who you are.

The start of your healing process is coming to peace where you are. When you can accept your circumstances without judgment, it becomes possible to quickly align yourself with what you want and where you want to be. In the example of the lady with the frozen shoulders, she did not recognize that her feelings about her mom had such an impact on her perception of her current circumstances. Until I did a recap of her own story about what was affecting her, she had not been able to form the connection. In a moment of inspiration, when she came to terms with her life in the present moment, she was able to see how much it was affected from an incident many decades ago.

Up until that moment, she did not have the tools or techniques to move beyond that feeling of the burden that life piled upon her. I conducted my exam, reflected upon her verbalized self-perceptions and performed the treatment, which gave her the helping hand to get over her obstacles.

From here we will address the toxins and nutrient deficiencies that came of the years of imbalance that her body had to adapt to. The pressure and tension in her body is now relieved because of the emotional shifts she has experienced. Her body is now wanting the resources that it needs to come back into balance. The resistance that she was carrying inside since she was six years old, caused problems that were accelerated over the last four years since the purchase of the franchise. Even though she had been eating healthy and teaching exercise classes, there was no amount of outside-in type of modality that could help her. No supplement, diet, body work or medication was fully effective.

However, since her breakthrough and awareness of her role in her condition, coupled with her new emotional vantage point of her life and circumstances, her body is ready to accept any resources it can utilize to accelerate healing. Prior to that, anything that she did to improve her health was an added responsibility or burden. But now her excitement is restored and she has a positive sense of the possibility for her own reasons for doing things, her own choices and the sense of ownership of her own life.

From this point, her work with me is geared towards rebalancing her physical structure and learning to use strategies and perspectives that reflect a life that is completely hers and is created by her own desires. Because most of her life, her body was used to supporting the energy of resistance to her natural desires, that is more the norm for her than giving into her own will. Her body became filled with tension and damage due to the pushing against effect that it had to maintain in order to support that resistance. We will continue to support her healing process until balance within her body, mind and emotions is restored.

The Energetic Shift

In western medicine, we are so used to addressing what presents physically in the body, without any regard for the mental, emotional and energetic components of it. For this reason, most treatments provide only temporary benefit and lackluster results. In the rare occasion, where a treatment results in a complete healing, the patient has somehow addressed the mental, emotional and energetic component on their own.

The energetic shift is like a train switching tracks. Unless there is a change, like a switching station on the railroad track allowing a train to get on the track to a new destination, there is no possibility of getting anywhere other than where you were originally headed. Until you switch tracks, anything that you do to accelerate your progress, simply gets you to where you're headed faster. And if you don't like where you're headed, you're not going to like the ride. But when you get on the right track, speeding up the journey gets you to where you want faster.

Remember. You are energy. You are more space than you are solid. Your body responds to your thoughts and emotions because they are energy. Your chronic thoughts and emotions hold your body at a standstill until you are able to shift them.

Until this time, your body continues to give you signals or symptoms in an attempt to guide you back into balance. Every time you don't get the message, your body sends you a new message. If you can't hear it, don't worry, it will get louder. Eventually you will make the shift. The question becomes how much time will you have left to enjoy the benefits of making the shift?

Chapter 5

Life Is a Mandelbrot

When people come into my office with a pain, symptom or disease, treating and getting rid of the presenting problem is obviously our goal. But we seem to have gone on quite a journey in the last four chapters, taking us from the focus on treating pain and symptoms alone to considering many more possible contributing factors.

In Chapter 1 we talked about symptoms being the story and the simple fact that they are signals from our body telling us that we are resisting the natural flow of life and there could be an easier way. We looked at the ways in which life is symbolic, in Chapter 2. Then in chapter 3 we discussed the concept of intention and right use-ness, what you are setting out to do and how to go about accomplishing that. In chapter 4 we looked at how everything in life is governed by a flow of energy and that we are energy.

In this chapter, I'd like to provide a scientific model that serves as evidence for the way I help my patients overcome their pain and symptoms forever. So you're probably wondering what a Mandelbrot is. Basically it is a fractal, which is a scientific equation that produces a repeating pattern that keeps elaborating in complexity and can be seen as a beautiful image that repeats as you zoom in or out. You will often see fractals as screensavers on computer monitors. I'm going to show you how this repeating pattern represents the complexity of the unfolding of your life.

Benoit Mandelbrot discovered the mathematical equations that produce these beautiful patterns in 1975, when he was studying the length of the coast of Britain. He explained them as geometrical shapes that continue to repeat. This repeating pattern creates a larger shape that is a replica of the smaller shape. These patterns were recognized before, but he was the first person to really describe it and study it with the use of computers. The power of computing allowed him to do thousands of equations in a few moments, enabling him to magnify the equation and play it out continuously and infinitely.

So how, you may be wondering, does this explain my symptoms and what does it have to do with my life? There are mathematical principles behind the feeling and expression of life. There are experiences that repeat in our lives. Different people may repeatedly fill the same role that keep playing over and over in your relationships. Situations may keep arising in your life no matter what you do. And you just keep on trying to change the situations but no matter what, different faces, different places, you always get the same outcome.

So the question is, what is the attraction that brings about or causes these repeating situations in your life? When you really look at your life, you may notice that the same kinds of people, similar relationship problems, identical financial problems, repetitive injuries, and other same old things keep showing up. Part of it is you, your environment, you're thinking and your physical process. All these levels are one and the same and whether they are within or around us, they need to be addressed. Particularly in the emotional realm.

I remember a time in my personal life when I was going through a lot and struggling. Things were getting worse and worse in a relationship I had with a woman. No matter what I tried, we could not seem to make it work easily.

One day when I was under a particular amount of emotional stress, I went for a run in the backwoods near the high school where I grew up. When I finished my run, I realized that I had lost my keys. It just seemed like nothing was working out. But I pulled myself together and figured that there must be some meaning to this.

At that moment, I realized that staying in this relationship was a constant effort. The same problem kept showing up time and again and the harder I tried to fix it, the worse it got. I knew at that point that I had to make a decision. I decided to end that relationship.

That decision changed the course of my life from that moment forward. I had already called my old high school to tell them that I had lost my keys nearby. The moment I came to terms with what I had to do, my phone rang. It was someone from the school calling to tell me that somebody had turned in my keys.

The moral of the story is that life is always giving you insights. It let's you know when things are going really well and it shows you when things are going down the wrong path. If you're on the wrong track and missed the signals, don't worry, they'll get louder. Losing my keys in the woods was a loud, inconvenient message. When I got the message, it was no longer needed and I got my keys back.

How to Start Recognizing Fractals in Your Life

These fractals can also be positive events, circumstances and life experiences, however, it is typically the problems that get our attention. To spot a fractal, it starts out as, "I have a problem in my life." To make it simpler, let's consider recognizing the problems in different levels. We will observe them from the physical body, emotions, thoughts and the overall connection and meaning.

Physical

The body and physical symptoms is as good a place as any to start, because it's with us wherever we go. It always has our attention. I'm going to show you how to observe it and use it to recognize repeating patterns in other places in your life.

Clues about where to start can be a part of your body that you keep injuring, pain that has been in one area for a long time or a chronic disease. Pain is a big motivator because it gets our attention and makes it difficult to focus on other things. It is very important to give respect to the pain and to welcome it as teacher or guide that will lead you to the answer. Ultimately, from this physical symptom, you want to develop your awareness so that you can investigate the feelings and the emotions behind it. This will lead you to the story that it tells.

For example I have a patient who has recurring foot pain. He always seems to stub his toe. While this started out as just a physical issue for him, it has been chronic and I know that all the different components of his life are tied into the root cause of this issue.

If we consider the fractal nature of this, the body part in pain is the alarm or the alert. It means you're on a path and there is a pattern that is continually unfolding. As long as you have that alarm, you're on the same path and that is why your life looks the way it does. Each component of life builds on other previous components. The big picture of your life looks a lot like the little pictures. The body part is just the start and a place to get your attention so that you look at the bigger picture of what you're creating. It leads into what you value, what you believe, what you hold onto and all the emotional baggage.

How to Use this in Your Body

Developing your awareness around your pain and symptoms is a powerful way for you to take an active role in the bigger picture of what your life looks like. I train my patients to develop a strong physical awareness. It's a self-reflection. I ask them to pay more attention to the part of their body that is hurting and giving them problems.

For example, with the fellow who keeps stubbing his toe and the chronic foot pain, I asked him to pay attention to his foot more. Until then, he had been trying to ignore it while still doing all the same things he had always done. Obviously, this did not work very well, because all his symptoms just kept getting worse. So I asked him to pay attention to the sensations that he was feeling in his foot but you can do this with any part of your body.

The Body Breathing Technique

Focus your breath and your attention on the specific body part that hurts. Let your mind relax and focus your breath on the area of discomfort. Bring attention to this area of your body. This will allow a message to be revealed. This is the message your body has been trying to tell you all along.

Observing your inward self will give you a break from all the mental chatter and jog your memory. The hurting body area will begin to project an internal movie onto your thoughts and at this point, memories, images, feelings and sounds may come up as well. This is showing you a piece of the puzzle and an answer to why the pains and health problems are there in the first place. At first this may just reveal the most current and important layer.

The Emotional Level

When you practice the body breathing technique, you will experience your emotions becoming active. You need to be able to detach a bit from what you experience. Emotions can have a tendency to hijack you and pull you right into the story. The feelings and emotions may be related to the injury or they may trigger memories or even a song. If you sit with the emotions and allow yourself to experience them, you can get to the inside and the aha then can come.

Be careful not to get reabsorbed into the emotional experience and play out the whole scene. You can get overwhelmed and pulled into the same old emotional patterns. Step away and play the observer. This way you will not get pulled into the story that is associated with the injured body part and the emotions.

Anger for example, is a powerful emotion that wells up inside you. It is very common for the feeling to have a belief or thinking pattern associated with it. The emotional trigger quickly pulls us into a story and we no longer experience the reality that we desire. We get pulled into the story that the anger is anchored to. When you do the body breathing technique and you focus your awareness on the location of pain, it is important to see the pain and the emotions as what they are, a signal, not the story that you have created around them.

The pain or emotional trigger is like an app on your phone. When you run the app, it plays the story the way it's supposed to and accesses the physical, emotional, mental and energetic connections associated with that injury. While the app is running, you stay entertained and absorbed in the story without really having the present moment experience right around you. You end up thinking that what is playing out in the app is reality.

The true reality is something else. It's what is happening in your body, what's happening around you and knowing that you can develope a new perspective on it anytime you want. The app will always do the same thing but if you change your perspective, it's like reprogramming the app. All of a sudden you get a whole new experience of the physical, emotional, mental and energetic levels of life.

Most people's lives are repeating patterns that keep

them frustrated and stuck. The apps that are running them, have physical, and emotional, or mental triggers that play unsupportive and unfulfilling stories. These stories build upon each other and spiral into the big picture of the life they live. It's painful and it's not pretty.

The good news is, that acknowledging and bringing awareness to the physical sensations and the emotions associated with them, is the first step in recognizing the patterns that are creating your life. This causes a shift in consciousness that is critical to understanding how something in your life may be affecting you. This point is pivotal in changing the fractal pattern that emerges from here. You are in essence, changing your story, which changes the pattern in which your life unfolds. It creates a whole new picture.

The Mental Level

Our thoughts direct our attention and cause us to focus on the circumstances and events around us in a particular way. They assign meaning to things that actually have no meaning and they create the story of how life works for us. When we let this happen without direction, we end up creating our reality unconsciously. If we are not careful about the thoughts we let into our minds, unsupportive thoughts get in there and grow like weeds.

Once we can observe the pain and the emotions for what they are, we can start to observe the beliefs and thinking patterns associated with them. If you stick with the body breathing method as the observer, this will allow you to see the story behind the pain and emotion.

Many of the beliefs and thinking patterns are probably not even yours. They were probably imposed on you or modeled by you from your parents, siblings, friends, caretakers and teachers around you. Many of them were observed and practiced since you were a young child. The awareness of our stories helps us to understand where we came from. It also helps us to chart a course for where we are going.

The Story

When we observe our story, we can see how deeply entrenched it is in all the patterns that repeat in our lives. We play different roles in the story in different circumstances. Sometimes we may be victims, other times heroes and we may even play the villain. This is very general but it's a theme that we even observe in our entertainment. The story we hold onto is at its core, from our childhood or young adulthood. Our beliefs and values are shaped by this story and they tend to play out unknowingly. Some of them help us and many of them cause us to sabotage what we really want. Our stories encourage our thought process and they can affect us in a positive or a detrimental way. They're on both sides of the coin.

You can use this awareness and choose to consciously shape your story. You are in effect changing the Mandelbrot of your life when you do this. We each are our own Mandelbrot. We are part of the same equations but just one of the infinite permutations. Any permutation from any point can be possible. We start out with a certain repeating pattern that can continue infinitely and unchangingly. As we make decisions and choices, we add new factors to the equation and a new avenue emerges. A new limb grows from the tree.

My own personal philosophy is that we all have infinite potential and multiple destinies. As we make decisions, we change our course and begin to trend towards specific destinies. If you feel that you are moving into the wrong destiny, make the decision to change it. Instead of feeling held back just take that step forward. That one step introduces you to new possibility and a new destiny.

In the example of the fellow with the foot pain, the story was centered around self-worth. The pain would remind him of physical injuries that occurred in stressful times of his life. It would bring up the emotions of frustration and the inability to get his own way. He was caught up in a story of thinking that his way was the right way. When things did not go his way, he had to look for a reason why. The answer was always, "It must be me and I'm not worth it." This figuratively put a nail in his foot and he did not move forward from there.

He developed the rock solid conclusion that, "I'm not worth it." Life was always colored that way and that's how his life kept playing out for many years. In all his experiences, he kept attracting situations where, whenever things got good, he would hit the glass ceiling. In his relationships, he could not commit. He would sabotage it and the relationship would break up. In his career, he was never holding down a long-term job and work was always causing him strife. In his personal life, when playing on sports teams, the team would not like his attitude. He was always trying to call the shots, but he was not the leader.

As he has been practicing his awareness around the pain in his foot and working with the body breathing technique, a lot of his meaning that has been running his life has been revealed to him. He has become much more at peace with himself and his life. The pain is going away and injuries are not recurring. He is experiencing much more positive emotions and his relationships are getting better. He has much more motivation in life and he describes the feeling as an accumulation of positivity. This has happened progressively over the last six months but it has added up into a major shift.

He has stopped being his own worst enemy. His awareness has opened him up to new decisions in every moment. Each new decision shifts him into a new permutation of the equation for his life. Each time he does this, a deeper and more beautiful pattern emerges and the picture of his overall life changes shape. He has become a conscious creator in life.

Every patient who has an ongoing issue of some sort can use this form of awareness to gain insight into the issue. The issue is the sign that is telling them to pay attention to something that they believe about themselves. It's always an inside job and with that knowledge, it becomes empowering. There is always something that you can do for yourself and you can accomplish this faster with the help of a mentor. This is the role that I play my practice. It's an honor to help my patients develop this awareness so that they can heal their issues once and for all.

Chapter 6

Stop Being Your Own Worst Enemy and Become Your Biggest Ally

"Whether you think you can or you can't, you're right."
— Henry Ford

By this point, you may have gathered that, how you think and feel, has a big impact on the sensations in your body. It's all a matter of awareness and perception. Life is a matter of perspective and whether you have a good or bad day, has to do with the the way you choose to see events and circumstances. You have the power to choose.

I would have to say, that taking responsibility for and being discerning in the thoughts you think are the two biggest things you can do to impact the quality of your life. In fact, if you were diligent in doing so, you would only be experiencing the good things that you want in your life and your body. I would probably have to find myself a new job.

I don't have any concerns about being put out of business though, because I know it takes dedication and practice to keep your thoughts focused on what you want in every given situation. We've been trained a certain way so long it's easy to get distracted and caught up in things that we don't like. For this reason, I know that I will always have a role in helping people learn how to manage their thoughts and emotions to keep their lives happy and their bodies healthy.

Inevitably, people come to me because they are experiencing pain in some part of their body. They keep coming back and refer their friends because I'm good at helping them relieve this pain and live happier and more comfortable lives. The reason I am so successful with this, is because whenever we have a location of pain, I know that there is an area of life, a belief, or connection to this spot that is out of balance.

Does Pain Mean that I'm Being My Own Worst Enemy?

Just because you have pain, does not mean that you're being your own worst enemy. However, oftentimes, we do discover that for many people, this is the case. In every circumstance, pain brings you to a point of decision about your next step. Sometimes we make this next step consciously and other times we default to what we've always done.

So in essence, pain guides you to become your own biggest ally. If every time we experienced pain, be it physical, emotional or mental, we stopped and asked ourselves, "What decision could I make right now that is in the best interest of myself and all involved," we would find ourselves creating a very happy life.

For most people, however, pain is considered something that needs to be taken care of, ignored and eliminated. We go to great lengths to do this and in doing so, we keep our focus in the wrong place. Most efforts go into treating, numbing or relieving this pain. There is little attention about the cuases to why we take certain actions that could make our lives happier and healthier.

How then, can we start using pain as the guide to understand how we can be our own biggest ally? Before I share how to do this, let me further clarify this concept with an example of a patient that I am working with.

Sally, a 41-year-old woman came in to see me with neck pain, right shoulder pain and headaches. The pain had come on following a motor vehicle accident. She's a very successful and driven women with a PhD. She has the typical Type A personality.

When I did my exam, the area that I found to be causing her problems, was not what she would have expected. In order to unlock this pattern, I found that I needed to go to her wrist. To achieve true healing, we can't reduce the body to the sum of its parts. There are connections everywhere and as you know, the hand bone is connected to the wrist bone, the wrist bone is connected to the arm bone and so on.

When I adjusted her wrist, it unlocked the shoulder pain and she got instant relief in her neck. Her headache went away as well.

A week later, when she came in for a follow up appointment, all the pain had returned. I asked her to tell me about how the symptoms resurfaced and she told me that it happened on Monday night. So I asked her what had happened that evening. She stated a number of things but also told me about an old boyfriend of hers who had called, asking for a professional reference. She was very surprised by the call. Upon further questioning, she also mentioned that she felt badly about the end of that relationship because she had treated him harshly. She felt that she had put more energy into her career than she had put into her time with him.

On reflection, she realized that she had matured in this area and now that she was in the beginning stages of a new relationship, she was concerned about balancing her work with her personal life. She was afraid that she would treat the new guy just like the old guy.

I knew that there had to be a belief or some mental/emotional component to the spot that would release this pain. I just needed to do some more testing to find out what it was. In passing, I dropped a comment about how we tend to treat the people closest to us the same way that we treat ourselves. This rang true for her.

One powerful technique that I use to determine the contributing factors to a person's pain, is applied kinesiology (AK). In this technique, we test for a reflex response in the body, sort of like the knee-jerk response that your family doctor tests with the little rubber hammer. I use that reflex to determine the body's response to various stimuli. One such reflex involves testing the strength of a muscle. When we find an offending stimulus, the muscle will test weak. When we apply the proper correction, the muscle should test strong in the presence of the offending stimulus.

My protocol is to first go through a set of physical stimuli, to see how the body responds. We then move onto testing toxins and nutritional components, to see if these factors are involved in a person's complaint. If I still don't have the answer, I move onto emotional and mental stimuli. I actually have the patient look at a list of different words and say them aloud as I test. In Sally's case, the word that made her test strong was "kindness."

The moment I said kindness, she realized that she had a belief that, in order to motivate herself to get things done, she needed to be aggressive. She had very harsh internal language and was always judging and critiquing herself.

This realization gave her a lot of clarity about the next steps that she needed to take. By the end of the session, the fogginess she was experiencing with her headache had lifted and she felt a sense of peace and balance. She could now see that she could motivate herself with kindness and that this could be the driving force in her new relationship as well.

Sally had been able to achieve a certain level of career success with her previous strategy of motivation, however, it came at a great cost to her. In fact, she had to ask herself if it was really worth it. Understanding how this belief was running her life set her free. She and I are now working through all the areas in her life where she has been her own worst enemy. Using her body as a guide, she is learning to be her biggest ally.

Recognize Where You are Your Own Worst Enemy

You can train yourself to see when your thoughts and beliefs are not supportive. This is a very important skill to develop and it is critical to living a happy, healthy and successful life. At first, it may seem like all you notice is negativity, but trust me, this is an incredible first step.

You want to start observing yourself in automatic behavior that brings on strong emotions like frustration, anger and short temperedness. Pay attention to how you react when things don't go your way and to how you speak to the people who are closest to you.

It is very common to have this come up with your parents or your spouse. I used to find myself very angry with my parents for no reason. I knew it was irrational and I could not understand where these emotions came from. If anyone else did what they were doing, it would not bother me at all. With my partner, this would come up when we are both tired after a long workday. There would be no filter and we would say things to each other that we would never say to a stranger.

The moment that I realized how much I was doing this, I was very grateful. I knew that this had to stop. I also gained the insight that my behavior towards them was simply a reflection of the way I was treating myself. How could I ever thrive when I was being so hard on myself? I would not be this mean to my enemies.

Getting to this point of realization and having the insight that you want to treat yourself better, is a moment of healing. This allows you to become more mature. You can start to shift your behavior and make it more congruent with the energy and the idea of what love is.

Internal Indicators

When we experience situations or circumstances in the present, past or future, our body becomes involved in the energy of the experience. We can become aware of how our body participates by paying attention to internal indicators. This means noticing sensations in your body.

When you are thinking about an experience that happened today or 20 years ago, your body begins to stimulate emotions and feelings connected to the event. You will want to learn how to describe them, by sensing them and view them. This is how you discover the indicators associated with the root experience that cause pattern behaviors or experiences that tend to repeat in your life. You will be able to uncover thoughts, memories, events and perspectives, some that don't support you, block you and that can cause you to hold onto the future or past.

Learning to sense these indicators works in both positive and negative ways. It is very easy to feel positivity around a vacation. Just think of your favorite vacation spot, be it the beach, a mountain or river. When we experience negativity, we tend to want to get away from it. We have been taught not to notice it or to avoid it altogether. We may take pills, stuff ourselves with food, use alcohol or smoke cigarettes. We try to override the sensations, by stimulating the body with something external.

These indicators hold a wealth of information for you. Paying attention to them and developing your awareness of them, will help you find the parts of your body that are associated with unsupportive patterns. This is a pivotal step in healing your body and making a shift in your life that brings you more joy and happiness.

Turn your attention inward and start to describe the sensations that you notice. Not the emotions but the feeling that you experience in a body part. Ask yourself if it is heavy or light, dense or expansive, smooth or rough. It may be fiery or watery. It could be flowing or backed up. This is your own self-assessment. You're not looking for pain, just a sensation, a description. If you do experience pain, stay with it and see what sensations are beyond it.

Discover Key Areas in Your Body with the Body Breathing Technique

When to Use this Technique:

This is a technique that you will want to use when you experience negative emotion. If you're driving home and you just can't wait have that glass of wine, that's a good indicator. Anytime that there are feelings that you would just prefer to avoid, it's a good time to tune in and pay attention.

Just the fact that you are knowing that you are having a negative feeling is a huge step. It is called awareness. When my patients start noticing and reporting these things, I tell them it is a huge celebration.

You can use the body breathing technique to discover where in the body that negative feeling is being held. Every emotion has an association with a particular part of your body. When there are patterns of emotion that you would like to change, it is very useful to find the associated body part.

How to Find "the Spot"

Clear some time and space for yourself so that you can be fully present, without being disturbed. Close your eyes and focus on your breath. Notice how the breath is happening to you and within you. Once you have focused on your breath, bring your attention to your toes. Move the breath into your toes as move your awareness there. Feel the sensations.

Next, bring your awareness upward and into your foot. Become aware of the feelings there. Notice your socks if you're wearing them and feel the pressure they exert. Once you've gained a deeper sense of the feet, move up the body to the ankles, the calves, the shins and the knees. Work your way from the bottom of your body to the top, taking time to pause at each new location and feel the tensions, pressures and sensations that may be present.

Some people find it helpful imagining that they have stepped into a hula hoop, that moves up their body and scans it as it passes. One or more locations will have a dense or heavy sensation, that feels different from the rest of the body.

Choose one of those dense areas and put your hands right on it. This will help you focus your thoughts in that one area. Focus your awareness into that area and breathe into it with attention.

In the beginning, it may take you a few minutes to complete this process. Work at being clear with the message that is being told to you by your body. As you gain experience, you will find that the story your body is telling you, will come up more rapidly.

How to Start Being Your Own Best Ally

Being your own best ally requires trust in yourself. The following process may seem a bit ambiguous but know that it doesn't have to work perfectly to be working right. Discovering what the story is, begins with knowing you only have part of the story figured out. Essentially, you have a single clue. In reality, what you have, are parts of the story coupled with a knowing, that any information that shows up, gets you on the right track.

In any given event, there are infinite perceptions you can have. The most important thing to consider is whether there is a better emotion that could improve the experience of the situation. What change in perception, feeling or attitude would be beneficial?

When you do this, a doorway opens. The story begins to break down and the search for a new meaning begins. Essentially, we are waiting for the brain to have an aha. When we ponder like this, the thinking part of the brain realizes that the current view is incomplete and it will begin looking for a better way to see things. Give yourself permission to shift, change or evolve an experience. The mind will go to work attempting to figure that out.

For me personally, the best way is to sit quietly, with the intention of positively evolving myself and finding a better way to handle this situation. This is accomplished by asking myself questions. Questions allow the meaning of an event to be re-defined. Once the Aha happens, I like to ask what new action can be taken to handle this situation with my new perception?

When you give the brain a problem, it will look for a

solution until it finds one. From there you will see a new behavior patterns emerging.

Ask Yourself Better Questions

Whenever we are interpreting a situation, the brain does so by asking questions. It asks questions like, "What's going on here," or "Have I seen this before?" Oftentimes, the questions that we ask are habitual and they pull up the same old answers. We accept the results we get as law and go no further. We continually act the same old way that we have always acted. This can severely limit our potential to experience joy. This is compounded by the fact that we often ask ourselves disempowering questions like, "Why am I so stupid?" You just can't win with any answer to that question.

A better question would be, "How can I be smarter and get a better result here?" Now the brain has a chance to find an answer that is empowering to you. And you can keep elevating the consciousness of the question you ask. You could ask, "How could I find an even better solution to this problem than I did last time?" If you always ask questions in a positive nature, your brain will continually seek out more and more supportive answers. Your job is to keep developing better quality questions.

Once you ask one good question, you start to get access to better questions. You begin to attract more nuances, details or specifics that you want to include in your questions. As you ask higher quality questions, it is as though you climb higher up flights of stairs, leading to more highly evolved answers.

How Do You Know if It's Working?

Working with a process like this is very subjective. The answers are very subjective as well. Don't ask yourself whether or not you're doing this right. Simply decide that you are going to get what you need.

In many cases, the aha is enough. You have gained the enlightenment. You notice your energy return. You feel more positive and ready to take on the day. From this state of mind, new options and choices will present themselves and you'll find yourself taking actions and making decisions that you never thought of before.

On the other hand, the insight or awareness may only be half the job. If there is a deep emotion that is stuck, the correlating part of the body is likely stuck as well. This is the case with most people that come to my office with their neck or back all locked up. If that spot in the body remains locked up, the emotion associated with it will always come back. The pattern that you are stuck in, is attached to the stuckness in your body.

Recall the lady from chapter 4 with the double frozen shoulders. The first week after I saw her she was doing great. The second week we only worked on the physical manifestation of the problem. She emailed me later in the week to tell me that the shoulder pain had returned. This told me that something deeper within her was coming to the surface. We had cleared the first layers, which had provided temporary relief, but had allowed subsequent layers to surface. This became our new area of focus for healing.

In the first visit, she discovered her perspective of, "life is piling up on me" and the physical layer of pain had cleared up. This allowed access to a deeper, more core issue that we could not get to on that first visit.

She had the "mom syndrome". She took on other people's problems. This had to do with her belief that, "other people can't solve their own problems." This issue was surfacing because we were able to clear the physical patterns associated with her first issue.

In order for her to heal, we had to find the core belief that would help her body release the stuck pattern. We needed to create a new perception in the situation, combined with the physical restructuring of her body so that she could move forward.

My role is to help her identify her own solution. It is not to give her a solution. I want her to come up with the new belief that is supportive of her self and others.

In my office, I offer people numerous ways to develop this awareness of stuck patterns in their life and stuck parts of their body. I use many techniques to guide people and I teach tools like emotional freedom technique (EFT) also known as tapping. If you are interested in learning more, please call my office to find out the date of my next workshop or visit my webpage at www.DrKevinG.com and read the blog.

Recognizing unsupportive patterns and beliefs is life changing. Just knowing that you are being your own biggest enemy is a huge awareness. Once you know this, you can begin the process of changing these patterns and beliefs. Becoming your own biggest ally helps you to change your story and change your life.

Chapter 7

The Amazing Power of Changing Your Beliefs About How You Heal

We have already discussed the importance of mind-set in how our life, health and happiness unfolds. I think it is very important to address the significance of beliefs in how people heal. The many hours of professional level training I've had access to, participated in and applied in my own life has clearly demonstrated to me the importance of belief.

Our beliefs shape our reality. They dictate what can and what cannot happen. The question is, where did those beliefs come from? Many of the beliefs that we have are not our own. They have been taught to us from a very young age, by our parents, teachers and social norms. They are cultural and reflect our societal viewpoints.

What is your belief about healing and how is it affecting the vibrancy of the health you enjoy? If you're living in the western world, I would guess that much of your experience is guided by the western philosophy of health. There are a few prevalent beliefs. We have thoughts about aging and the decline of our bodies and expectations of how we will function over time. We are very used to being told that we are just going to have to live with things and that this is as good as it gets.

I would like to propose that you can have a very different experience, if you just bring some awareness to the thoughts you think about your own health and the actions you take to become healthy. I want to show you how much more is possible and that you can heal and enjoy a better quality of life, no matter what your starting point.

Let's start with why anyone goes to a health professional. When we seek help, it is because we can't figure out anything else to do on our own. We are usually experiencing a problem and are frustrated. We don't know how to fix it or where to turn. At some point we decide that it is just too much and we make the call for help.

Who you call depends on your mindset about the path you want to take. You may decide to do something medically oriented or you may choose a more holistic route. The practitioner that you choose will dictate the solutions that you will be offered. You will get their opinions about your problem based on their experience, knowledge and expertise.

If you go to a medical practitioner, you will tend to get pharmaceutical or surgically oriented answers. You will likely go through a series of tests to determine what is wrong and then your practitioner will make a diagnosis. They will then prescribe a medication or recommend a procedure to try to correct the problem. When you get sick, the medical professional believes that something has gone wrong in your body and they need to fix it.

If you go to a holistic practitioner, you will get answers that are more geared towards you as a person. They will be looking at how you have gotten out of balance and why. The problem that you come to them with, is viewed as a signal that there is something out of balance that you need to address. Again, based on their expertise and experience, they will recommend a course of action to correct what they believe the imbalance to be. It maybe something to do with physical alignment if you see a chiropractor, nutritional supplements if you see a nutritionist or your chakras if you see a reiki practitioner.

Choosing your practitioner is like choosing a restaurant. When you choose a place to eat, you know that the meal that you will get will depend on the type of restaurant you go to. You won't get a fine dining experience at a fast food restaurant and an Indian restaurant won't serve you pizza. You make your choice of restaurant with the expectation of the type of meal you expect to get.

When you choose the medical route, the expectation is that you will get tests, medications and possibly surgery. Most people choose the medical path because that's what they have always done. People believe that they are broken and sick. They accept the outcomes because that's all they know. They never really question what beliefs they are subscribing to by doing this.

Do you really believe that you were born with too many body parts and that some need to be cut out for you to be healthy? Does your health decline because you don't have enough drugs or medication in it? If you believe these things to be true, then it would make sense that removing parts of your body and filling yourself up with drugs will help.

When you choose the holistic route, it is likely that you believe that your body needs nutrients that are found in nature. There is a balance that needs to be established physically, emotionally, mentally and hormonally to remain healthy. Your practitioner is going to look at the aspects of balance within you to see what you are doing that has upset the balance. The expectation here is that you will get adjustments, nutritional supplements, exercises and or practices to help bring you back into balance.

In chapter 1, we discussed the fact that symptoms are a signal or a warning that tell us something is wrong. This is my viewpoint as a chiropractor and holistic practitioner. When the check engine light comes on in your car, you check the engine to make sure that you aren't going to burn it out. You don't decide that the light is annoying and distracting and put tape over it so it stops bothering you. This is very dangerous. In my opinion, treating a symptom so that it stops bothering you, is like doing this.

However, when you go to a medical practitioner, because the symptom is disrupting your life, they apply their expertise to treat the symptom, because that is what they do. If you go see a surgeon, because you have low back pain, the only solution you can expect is surgery to fuse vertebrae, cut out disks or some kind of management until the problem gets bad enough to require surgery. That's the kind of restaurant they are and that's what they serve. It does not matter that 99% of the time, low back pain is happening because something else is out of alignment with that person. Regardless of whether it is physical, mental or emotional, when you see a surgeon, the course of action is surgery.

When part of your body wears out, you need to ask why. Is it because of age? If that were the case, why isn't your whole body wearing out at the same rate? It is very common to find degeneration in one or two vertebrae in the spine, while the rest are perfect. Even thinking that it's because of the things you do, like your job, demanding sports or sitting too long, is questionable. Are there other people who do the same things you do, that don't have the same problems you have?

We create a lot of problems for ourselves by believing that our body is broken or built for breaking down. Many people believe that the doctor knows everything. First of all, they don't. Second, the assumption that they know everything means that you know nothing. You give up your power over your own healing.

One of my patients, Jack, came in and told me that he blew out his back picking up his three-year-old niece. I understood that he got the symptoms after lifting the little girl but I wanted him to get a deeper understanding of the cause. It turns out that Jack is a HVAC professional and that he picks up heavy things every day. That week he was lifting heavy air conditioner units and getting into difficult positions. Why did it go out this week versus a different week?

People bend over and to lift things all the time. Why do some have pain while others don't? What other things are going on, creating a problem for them but not for the others? We need to shift our focus from viewing pain as a problem, to seeing it as an indicator or a warning light. This is one of the biggest beliefs to shift and when you do, it opens the door to a whole new realm of health possibilities.

Pain is a powerful motivator. We can tolerate pain, until it starts to disrupt our life enough, that we feel we need to do something about it. We find that the way we've been taken care of ourselves has limited benefit. Something physically, chemically or emotionally has gotten out of balance and we need to realign. The pain is the signal telling us to give our body what it needs to function and restore itself.

I find it very interesting when somebody goes for surgery. The doctor performs the surgery, fixes them up and when they wake up, tells them that the surgery was successful. They cut something out, put bones back together or sewed up tissues. Now the doctor tells them, that they need to rest and let nature take it's course. The doctor is basically telling them that they need to rely on their bodies own healing ability to finish the job. What if you started there in the first place?

The Middle Ground

What if we use pain and symptoms as a guide to find out what is out of balance? You can seek guidance from a practitioner who understands this perspective and will help you explore the reasons for the signals your body is giving you. Their assistance is a middle ground between your body's natural healing abilities and guiding you to trust in them, while helping you give your body what it needs to restore balance.

Consider the example of the a bank vault. There are two ways for a bank robber to get into it.

1. They can crack the combination, which is a subtle formula and a delicate dance

2. They can use dynamite to blast it open, which is more aggressive and destructive, but gets the job done

With method one, you can use the door multiple times, whereas with method two, the door is permanently altered and may never work again.

When I work with my patients, I like to use the first method. I find the combination of structural alignment, nutritional sufficiency, toxin elimination, and mental and emotional balance to unlock the door. When we get inside, we can find out what is out of balance and bring it back into harmony.

When people get drugs and surgery, they often find that they are not the same after. These interventions alter the body and limit its ability to heal fully. Because the original cause of the problem continues, it eventually overwhelms the drug or surgical solution and the problem returns. Most people don't want to go that route again or risk getting more damaging treatment. Using drugs and surgery can be like using dynamite to get the door open.

If you have gone the surgical route, you can still restore health. It is however, more complex, takes more work and you are dealing with limitations that have been physically imposed on you. But you don't have to live in pain and you can get your life back. This depends on which procedures were done, what was removed and the number of interventions you've had. Some people think that they are too far gone but I have found that this is never the case. These patients simply require dedication to their body's natural healing ability and time.

You may have believed one story and gone down that path for a long time. You basically went to the same restaurant and never questioned what you were served, even though you didn't enjoy it. But it's never too late to decide that you want a better experience and that you're going to a new restaurant.

You need to change your story. You need to believe that you have the power and that you are your own advocate. The doctor is there to make suggestions based on their perspectives but you know what is best for yourself. You are intelligent and you can make good decisions.

Innate Intelligence

Have you ever wondered what the difference is between a living, breathing human being and a corpse? They have all the same parts but there is something very different about them. That difference is the life energy that keeps a body vital, regenerating and healing. That life force or innate intelligence makes the difference between the living body thriving and the corpse basically rotting.

If you take a moment and appreciate a plant or a baby or even how your heartbeats and all your organs run automatically, you will be in awe. No one has to direct the multitude of functions that occur so that we can experience life. The innate intelligence in that plant, that baby and in you, is the expression of life, it creates well-being naturally. That is the purpose of innate intelligence. Can you imagine what would happen if you actually had to think about all the processes and functions in your body in order for it to work? You would not be able to focus on anything else and impossible to track all your responsibilities. It's a good thing your heart beats and you keep breathing all night.

Choosing the Right Professional

There is a time and place for every type of professional. I am very grateful for our medical system, for drugs and for surgery. If I were smashed up in an accident, I would not go to my chiropractor or my massage therapist for help first. I would want to be pumped full of life saving medications and handed over to the surgeons, so they can work their magic.

However, when I am looking for a way to go from healthy to healthier, I am not going to turn to a medical professional. That would be like asking the fire department to pump thousands of gallons of water into your house to prevent fires.

In times of crisis, we often need more significant interventions. But most of the time, we are not in crisis. The pain may feel like we're in crisis, but it is simply an alarm that has been getting louder and louder, to tell you to get back into balance. If you take care of things routinely, crises can be completely avoided and the alarms stay quiet.

To get the best results in your healing, you need to find a practitioner who can guide you to rebuild your trust in innate intelligence. You need someone who helps you to refocus your beliefs in a way that make you successful in achieving the health you want.

10 Beliefs that Disempower Healing

The most powerful thing that you can do to live a happy, healthy and vibrant life, is to make sure that all your beliefs support the health that you want. Unfortunately, most people that I encounter have many disempowering beliefs, that make them decline and get sicker with age. The following is a list of the 10 most common disempowering beliefs I encounter.

1. When you hit 40, it's all downhill
2. It's too difficult to learn something new, why try
3. There are no options
4. Change is bad and will mess something up
5. Failure means I'm finished
6. I'm nobody special
7. All germs are bad for you
8. It's not possible
9. Life has no meaning or purpose
10. A bad situation you're in is someone or something else's fault

10 Beliefs that Empower Healing

1. I love, accept and appreciate myself, just as I am
2. Relaxation, self care and meditation are important
3. I value the people around me

4. I can adapt easily to life's challenges

5. Physical activity is enjoyable

6. Having fun and pleasure is important

7. Life is full of beauty and optimism

8. I am resilient and self-reliable

9. Life can always be hopeful and helpful

10. I am willing to develop and cultivate myself and my life

The purpose of innate intelligence is to flow through you and create well-being. When we simply allow this to happen, we get health naturally. All it takes is the belief that this well-being is constantly flowing within us. As long as we don't block it and we give the body what it needs, we can continually get healthier and healthier. Use the list of 10 empowering beliefs above to create the health and happiness you want in your life.

Chapter 8

Change Your Story, Change Your Life

We talked a lot about beliefs in previous chapters. The beliefs that you hold will shape the quality and experiences of your life. There is a lot of power in making sure that your beliefs are supportive of what you want and what you want congruent with right use-ness. This chapter is all about focusing on and creating what you desire in life.

A belief is just a thought that you keep thinking. You may have been taught to think it but in essence, it is the story that you tell yourself over and over. The story of your life is a series of thoughts and beliefs that you repeatedly tell yourself and most people never think to change the script. The saddest thing is, most people don't really like their story.

The Roles We Play

Much of our story is made up by the different roles we play. We are characters in our own story and we assign our roles. We even assign others internal perceptions of ourselves and their potential beliefs, and we also assign what we represent to different things and different people. We create story and we play roles. These roles can be man, woman, brother, sister, husband, wife, employee, and employer and the list goes on and on. Each of these roles has a story to fulfill based on what you believe to be true about that role.

How we see ourselves in these roles can prevent our progress or launch us forward in life. While each of these roles has no meaning, we may have associated them as being positive or negative based on our experience. As we switch between our roles, sometimes we play the hero and sometimes we play the victim.

One of my favorite authors, Alberto Villoldo, is a PhD who worked in South America and has studied the shamanic rights and philosophies of ancient wise people. The opening quote in one of his books is really fitting here.

"We are what we think. All that we are arises out of our thought. With our thoughts, we make the world."—Buddha

Reading his book, "Courageous Dreaming" has caused me a lot of time in thought about the impact of my assigned roles and how I see myself in people's lives and healing. Much like what we see on TV and in the movies, our lives are a script in which we play the victim, the hero or the villain. And if you're sad, you're the victim and you need people to fill the other roles. There needs to be someone to bully you and someone to rescue you.

But if we shift our perspective to being a creator or the Hero, as Villoldo calls it, the bully becomes a challenge that makes us stronger and the rescuer becomes the coach or person who supports us. It's all a story of perspective of purpose in life.

Who are You Being?

One of my favorite classes, when I was studying chiropractic at Palmer Chiropractic College, was a course in geriatrics. One day, the professor brought in her hundred plus year-old mother. She was a member of the centenarian club and was accompanied by four or five other members. They all spoke to us of their thoughts on life. Each and everyone of them had an amazing sparkle in their eyes and so much enthusiasm in the way they told their stories.

You would think that these centenarians would all have impeccable diets and exercise regularly, however, some drank responsibly as they pleased and some had periods of smoking as well as various other habits of life. The difference was their attitude that everything in life happened to them in a good way. If they encountered a problem, there was always something to learn or gain. They could always find the silver lining in any situation.

Personally, I have experienced living from two viewpoints. I've had an extremely negative viewpoint where there is always a problem. I've also lived life with the perspective that there's always a solution or something good to find. We have the choice of being either of these people at any given time. If you take the time to ask yourself who you are being, it has a massive impact on your experience in any situation.

I spent much of my time in my teenage years focusing on the negative. In my mid 20s, I knew that I should be thinking and talking about the positive and that even negative situations had something to teach you. Life has a

way of continuing to bring you experiences when you have
something to learn from them. Over time, my perspective
shifted to seeing that life is beautiful and has meaning and
purpose. Even though it was not happening, that was my
practice. I had to get myself out of the mood state of anger
or depression. I wanted to raise my vibration and the regular emotions I was feeling. When I finally got the vibra-
tional state where I felt good more than not, it was like the
blinders came off. I was able to see different perspectives in
situations, giving me new ways to interact with people and
new solutions.

So much of the way that we interact with people and our
environment, has to do with the roles we play, that the TV,
movies, magazines and the media have taught us. People
around us fill various roles of our story and we respond with
automatic emotions which affect our surroundings. This experience guides me to become even more highly aware of
my thoughts and feelings. For example, my five month old
is like a canary in a coal mine. When I'm positive, she coos
happily and when I'm frustrated, she fusses and cries.

How we go about experiencing and perceiving events
in life, builds a pattern. Our previous experiences color our
expectations of how future situations will play out and create a groove or pattern of nerve fibers in our brain.

Are You Wired to Be Happy or Grumpy?

How we respond to situations is also a question of
our neurology. Our brain and nervous system gets wired
by the emotions we had during different experiences. I
often heard in school, "If they fired together, they wired

together." This means that if an experience stimulates your nervous system and you feel an emotion repeatedly, your brain and neurology will link the event with the feeling. You essentially become wired to have a particular emotion every time that event or similar event occurs. That emotion could be anger or joy. In any situation, you can effectively become wired to be happy, grumpy or anything in between.

This wiring is so powerful that, even remembering a particular situation can stimulate the components of your nervous system to release hormones, generate physiological responses and put you in an emotional state. Your body does not know if you are actually living the experience or just thinking about it. This is what keeps propagating the belief of "I'm not good enough", "I'm not worthy" or "I don't deserve this" in so many people. It's now in a groove.

Because the linking of emotions to a situation is so automatic, it can be a big challenge for people to change their story. It takes conscious awareness and a real desire to create a new outcome.

The reason for this, is that your brain wants to protect you from harmful situations. When you touch a hot stove, you withdraw your hand before you even feel the sensation. Your nervous system knows that it is best to pull you out of a dangerous situation before contemplating if too much damage is done. Unfortunately, when we experience a situation as harmful and associate negative emotions with it, our mind treats it like a hot stove and reacts which continually pulls us away, before we feel the pain. This wiring makes it difficult to create new associations. The emotion we experience keeps us locked in the story.

I had the pleasure of replacing one of my old stories just the other day. A venue had refused to host an event that I had been planning, because they did not agree with the viewpoint of the speaker. When I received the email from them, I got all fired up and felt like they were messing up my career. I had been having a great day until that moment. Then everything turned upside down. This change in attitude even affected how I spoke to my partner. I was taking my frustrations out on her and our baby got so upset that she didn't want me to hold her.

Fortunately, I stopped myself and decided that I did not want to feel like this. I apologized to my partner and went to sit outside. I told myself that I knew there was something good here for all involved and decided to let the emotions play themselves out. My brain began to look for the positive in the situation. After a few minutes of looking at the trees and squirrels, I had an aha. I started to relax and breathe again and was able to return having a happy and wonderful evening with my partner and our baby.

My old story had been that when people interfere with my plans, they are limiting or preventing me from excelling in my career. My new story is that these people and situations are guiding me to where my career needs to be. This subtle difference put me in the driver's seat and made me see the opportunities that were always there.

The very next day, I began discussions with a much larger venue that would be able to accommodate the demand for the speaker I was hosting. I was grateful that this situation happened and had guided me to step up and play at a bigger level.

What to Do When You Notice You're Having an Automatic Response

When we find ourselves in situations that cause us to react, it can be very difficult to notice what's happening. You may notice right away or it may take hours. When you become aware of this, just be happy that you have the opportunity to change.

Start with focusing your attention on what you sense within. Notice your stress response. Feel the adrenaline rush. Is your mind racing? Are your palms or your armpits sweaty? What is the mode of emotion in you? Is it firey, sad, depressed, overwhelmed or anxious? What is actually happening? Are you getting thrown into a spin because what you expected is not happening? Are you like a child throwing a tantrum? Is there a feeling of eruption within? Whatever you notice, start by being glad that you are noticing these sensations and doing this consciously to provide yourself with a gift of peace and wonderment.

Use the body breathing technique that we discussed in chapter 6. When something doesn't go my way, I like to use this technique to focus on my heart area. This is the area where my passion, my values, my loves and the things that I want in my life are kept. As you practice this exercise, notice the story that shows up for you.

Once I have identified the story that has been running my life in this situation, I like to use this Wayne Dyer exercise, to find a new and better story to replace it.

Say and feel to yourself:

I want to feel good.

I want to feel good about this.

I know there is something good here.
What is good about this?
Breathe deeply and repeat the statements until you feel at ease and/or have an aha moment.

This engages your brain to search for the side of life that is positive, solution-oriented and hero-oriented. The focus becomes finding a healthy way to get out of the negative emotional story, instead of resorting to eating, drinking or smoking to subdue the anger, fear and worry.

When you're driving your car and you get cut off, no matter how upset you get, how much you honk your horn, nothing is going to change the situation. Can you make a new choice to let that person go and thank God that everyone is safe? If so, you made a new choice to be at peace. You'll notice that when you arrive at your destination you are relaxed and ready rather than being frustrated.

This is how you tune into a new vibration. It's like changing the radio station to one that plays music you like instead of complaining about the bad music on the station that's always playing. You're creating a new story.

By living consciously and building on the positive, we attract more of what we want and everything seems to run more smoothly. We become a different person even though we are in the same situation. It takes on new meaning. Instead of battling the other players, we begin to move in the same direction and experience a greater ability to achieve the outcome we want. Whether this is in family, work or intimate relationship, there's a better flow of communication, resulting in more support, enjoyment, camaraderie and closeness. You'll find yourself wanting to be less selfish and more giving. You will see all areas of your life expand positively.

I see this in my practice all the time. There is an ease that starts developing in my patients and a wanting to do good for self and others. They develop an increased sense of certainty and personal empowerment. Their communication with the world is more centered, making it easier to operate and things tend to go their way.

When people start working with me, this transformation is immediate. This happens because we always talk about what is going on in their body and life. They tell me their story in their words and I listen to the language they use. This gives me a lot of insight into who they are being. As we create ease in their body, they get ease in their life.

I worked with a patient for a couple of months who grew up locally but had lived in California for a while. She had moved back into the home she grew up in and was living with her sister who is an alcoholic with considerable mental concerns. Upon arriving for the appointment she immediately told me, "I don't want to be there" and "I don't believe I can handle it." She gave me the mental root of her physical pain without my even asking. It was a story of self reliability. She believes she is stuck in her living environment and became stuck in her body.

During the treatment, I paused and asked her what she did want. I reframed her two statements and suggested that perhaps she wanted her own living arrangement and the confidence that she could handle any situation. I was able to listen to her words and read between the lines, thus clarifying her statement of what she did want. Body reflex testing showed that she was holding a stuck pattern that released when I adjusted her and she acknowledged her belief in herself. At the end of session she was calm, peaceful and optimistic about her next step as well as pain free.

Small changes in perspective lead to massive differences and how you live your life. A slight shift in direction results in a completely different destination. Simply applying the awareness described in this chapter will give you valuable information about automatic patterns in your life. Identifying your unsupportive beliefs and stories is so valuable and fulfilling. It may seem frustrating at first but just be happy when you catch yourself in a story you don't like. When you set your sights on what you do want, you can change your story and change your life.

Chapter 9

Life Is Perfect

I know it's a tall order to suggest that life is perfect, when there are things going on in the world that just don't make any sense. Some of the things that happened in your life in the last week may feel far from anything you would ever ask for. Bear with me. If anything from the last chapter resonated, maybe a slight shift in perspective could create a dramatic impact on how you feel about these events. If you can change your story to the point where you believe that everything is always working out for you, this new story will help you to see life's perfection.

So we may not be there yet, but give me a chance to build a case here. First I would like to introduce the concept of natural laws. A natural law is an observable rule that governs natural phenomena. It is undeniably, and indisputably true.

Gravity is a natural law. No matter how hard you try, in the presence of the Earth's gravity you will never fall up. Cause and effect is a natural law. Every cause, that is any situation or circumstance that occurs in a moment, will create an effect or an outcome related to it. And that effect or outcome becomes the cause of another effect. Attraction is a natural law. Every thought and emotion or action of a particular vibration will correspond with similar thoughts, emotions or actions. Your vibration attracts situations of similar vibrations. These natural laws are operating in your life and creating what you know to be true.

The results of the operation of natural laws in your life are exactly as they should be. What you see in your life is the result of natural laws that work time and time again. No matter how firmly you believe that if, this time, when you step off the side of the ledge, you will float up, gravity is going to take you down. If you bang your head on the wall, cause and effect will give you a headache. If you think the world is full of stupid people, the law of vibration dictates that even the smartest person will seem stupid to you.

These natural laws always work perfectly and will always yield results in keeping with their law. The results that these laws deliver, are always perfectly based on an individual's operation within the law. If someone jumps out of the plane falls to their death, the law of gravity yielded the perfect result. If that person uses a parachute and has a thrilling ride to the ground, their understanding of the law of gravity has allowed them to create the perfect result. Once you have an understanding of the natural laws, and you know how to operate within them, you begin to see that all outcomes are perfect. Whether they are what you want or what you don't want, that's your perception. They are still happening in perfection according to natural law.

So what, you maybe asking, does this have to do with my less-than-perfect-life? Well let me tell you. Knowledge or ignorance of the laws and whether you're adept at operating within them or not, does not matter. The laws are always operating perfectly. So what I am telling you is that, what is happening in your life right now and the results you're getting, are a perfect reflection of how you live and operate within these natural laws.

I work with people experiencing a lot of cause and effect every day. The symptoms that they complain about are the effect of a cause somewhere in their life. They observed the symptom and assume that it is the problem. They rarely consider that it is the result or effect of something else that they're not observing. Quite often people are oblivious to what brings the symptoms on. My job is to make them aware of their involvement in the cause.

Werner Karl Heisenberg was a German theoretical physicist and one of the key pioneers of quantum mechanics. In one of my favorite quotes, he says, "What we observe is not nature itself, but nature exposed to our method of questioning."

When something goes awry, the questions most people ask may be, "Why is this not working," or "Why is this not going my way?" The questions they do not ask could be as follows. How is this the perfect outcome of some action, decision or behavior that I was involved in? What thought, feeling or action, not yet observed can be done differently to provide the outcome I desire? Is my desired outcome in alignment with natural law?

Our observations about a situation or circumstance are not necessarily the facts, rather the interpretation our mind has of the question it is asking. Recall the list of the empowering and disempowering beliefs from chapter 7. The questions that we ask in any given situation reflect our beliefs and dictate how our mind searches for an answer.

Many things existed before humans had a means of observing and describing them. Primitive cultures would have observed phenomena like someone falling ill and dying and tried to correlate it to something. They may have associated the death with the fact that the person went into a forbidden area, where anyone who entered fell ill. They may have concluded that the place was cursed or that the person had angered the gods. Thousands of years later, when technology has evolved to a sufficient level, perhaps it is discovered that area is highly radioactive.

X-rays were discovered in the 1900s. The frequency of this type of energy was always present but our technology and thinking has matured to a place where we could discover and utilize them. Infrared and gamma ray technology has also worked this way. Just because we did not have a way of describing them, did not mean that they did not exist. We were still subject to their effects. So those poor humans that went into the forbidden area were simply subject to the effect of gamma radiation. The radiation was the cause of them falling ill.

The same is true for bacteria, and their presence in the cause of certain illnesses. They may have thought they were cursed and that everyone was dying from a plague. While today, with our knowledge of disease and germ theory, we know that with proper sanitation and a fully working immune system, these things simply do not occur.

When people are going about life and there is pain, a

feeling they don't like or something that is not going their way, they need to delineate between their personal beliefs about their experience and the objective or universal truths that governs them. Our personal beliefs are based on our own experience or what we have come to know. But in many cases, our perspective of the situation is skewed and may be false.

When people come into my office, they usually have a pain in some part of their body. As we have a conversation about the pain, they also tell me the stories that come with the pain. As I dig deeper, I ask them about challenges in their life that I consider to be related in their story. Inevitably a phrase will pop out of their mouth that shows me exactly where their belief has been limited or their expectation is negative. I often learned that they are observing something through a particular lens or story that is creating their result or outcome. Until they develop the awareness of the impact of their story, they associate their outcome to something other than themselves.

If we do in fact believe that life is perfect and that natural laws are yielding the perfect result, based on our operation within them, we can look at our results and ask new and better questions. We can take the experience and look for what is good and what there is for me to learn. When you work through a problem with this idea, another perspective shows up and you see that this challenge is here for your greatest good to grow.

But What if Life Does Not Feel Perfect?

When life does not look or feel perfect, it means that

you are out of alignment with your authentic self. You are out of alignment with natural law. There is a result that is happening because of some natural cause and effect. We are doing something to create it, yet we do not understand our role in it. We create stories about why this is happening or what it means based on our interpretation. We do not consider the objective facts or the thoughts, behaviors and actions we have taken that have a natural result of creating the perfection we are experiencing.

It is okay to feel this way. When we wake up to the fact that life is perfect but that we are not experiencing it as such, we have a golden opportunity. We know that we are out of alignment with our authentic self and that all we need to do is let go of a false story and act to realign with a better one.

Life Is Perfect. Big Deal. What Do I Do with This?

When you're frustrated and have the opinion that something is not perfect, start by just being happy that you realized this. Tell yourself that you are being guided to find a better way to see the situation. One that supports your well-being. Then it's time to question your own belief of your side of the story.

Natural laws are always present. They are binding, regardless of your belief or understanding. Gravity does not care if you are in a good or bad mood. Whether or not you believe you can walk on air, once you step off the cliff, gravity will take you down.

It always works. Cause and effect. The only factor to

consider is the time between the cause and the effect. If I like to speed, it may not happen right away, but eventually a police officer will catch me and give me a ticket.

Whether you are in pain, you don't like the way you feel or you're not happy with the situation you are in, you want to identify the cause. What actions, behaviors or beliefs are out of balance with your authentic self? Or, "How can I be more in balance with my authentic self?" When you ask yourself these questions, you will get an answer. Whatever answer you get, take action to improve it, this will set into motion more causes and effects. Keep using this guidance and adjusting what is out of balance and eventually there will be no reason for the pain to be there.

I had a patient that I've been treating for headaches. He would come in with his head hurting, I would do the adjustment, he'd feel better, shake my hand and leave. Two weeks later the headache would be back and we would go through the same cycle.

This continued to happen until one day, I asked him what he thought was causing it. He did not know. I asked him to walk me through his day and he did. At one point he recalled a stressful phone call. As soon as he brought this up, he hit himself in the forehead with his fist. I asked him if he realized what had just happened. He was oblivious. When I pointed out that he'd basically punched himself in the head, he woke up to all the times he had done this and how silly this habit was.

Further discussion around this behavior caused him to reveal that he would would get very stressed in situations that involved his work life. This had come from his belief that work was difficult and full of problems, a pattern that was passed on from his parents. When things got difficult or when he was a problem child, his parents would smack him on the head. The cascade of events that led to his head-ache started with a thought which lead to a behavior of hitting his own head, that led to the effect of his head hurting. The headache was the perfection that was able to bring his awareness to an unsupportive belief system, thought process and associated action.

Another client of mine had been frustrated by a recurring yeast infection for many years. She had been to multiple doctors, naturopaths and homeopaths and got lacklustre results. I have been working with her for years to address a number of other health issues. During that time I had also come to know a lot about her life, relationship and living environment.

Some advanced applied kinesiology training prompted me to test her for molds. She had already been taking a number of medications for yeast that would work only temporarily. This was puzzling me because I knew that there were molds causing the yeast infection but I did not know what was causing the mold to persist in her system. We always seemed to find the right remedy for her in my office but once she went home and came back, the potency of the remedy would be deactivated. This led me to testing air samples from her home.

Immediately we discovered that the air in her house was polluting her remedy. Multiple leaking water episodes were damaging the ceilings, resulting in continual mold growth.

This caused the infection, however, I knew that there

was yet another underlying cause. She and her husband had had many explosive fights over the years. Lots of tense emotions occurred in those moments. Because of the behavior of this type of communication, their house matched the energy. The house, a symbol of their relationship, leaked from the pipes and toilet. Interestingly enough, the symbolism associated with emotional feelings is water. It can be related to feelings of anxiety, terror, panic, frustration and fear.

In getting this lady to communicate clearly with her husband about her needs so she could reach an agreement with him about cleaning up their environment, she is making progress with her health. Now it's a question of helping her husband heal the explosive anger.

There is no accident to anything that exists in your life now. When you know that life is perfect, you can observe the conditions in your life and ask yourself what thoughts, feelings, behaviors and actions you have that may have contributed to this. You may just need some guidance to look at what's happening in your life. We often get into a groove or a way of being that is difficult to shift. Uncomfortable or undesirable conditions in our lives are great motivators for prompting big shifts.

This happens to everyone. Even though I'm a chiropractor, I can't adjust myself. I have to go to another chiropractor to get the complete workup, because sometimes I can not see through my own patterns. It is just so ingrained in us and foundational to who we are, that our logical brain can not reason it out.

I love this quote from Stephen Covey portraying the

viewpoint of a very prominent public figure during the time before cars were popular. "The horse and buggy is here to stay and the automobile is just a fashion."

People have such a hard time accepting change. They can't handle the shift so they deny it. The Germans argued with the Wright brothers for five years after they had been flying. They said it was not possible to fly.

When the gas light comes on in your car, you don't stick a happy face on the gas gauge and expect positive thinking to make it better. You go to the gas station. However when we experience symptoms in our body or something we don't like is happening in our lives, we do attempt to use this logic. We take an advil, run away or have a drink. We'd love to stick a happy face on it and just ignore the problem.

So How Do You Embrace the Perfection?

The joy really is in the journey. All our experiences are happening to guide us to make choices that fulfill our destiny and purpose in life. If you can subscribe to the idea that life is perfect, you begin to see the conditions as they are and question the meaning that you have placed on them.

I really like to apply the Wayne Dyer exercise in my life so I can see it's perfection. When I am trying to sort out a situation in my life, I make the following statements:

> I want to feel good about this.
> There is something good here for me to learn.
> I want to feel good about this scenario.
> What is good here?

This helps to shift the mind and allows us to take new

action. A simple change in perspective can lead to a small change in behavior. This one small change can shift the course of your life.

When I'm working with my patients, I am constantly observing how their body changes posture and shape as they explain the conditions that are affecting their lives. Different emotions involve different amounts of tension and positions of the body. As they tell me their story, their body tells me the truth. I know when the life they are living is not in alignment with their authentic selves.

After my assessment, I perform a treatment. The adjustment and other therapies I use are to support their body's release of interference so everything works well and reorients to better alignment . The result is the person standing and feeling tall, steady, light and flowing. They feel inspired, happy and relieved. I send them on their way with the new clarity and instructions to look upon their lives with new eyes.

If you have a problem, know that it is perfect. The problem is there to prompt you to move forward. Something you're doing, thinking or believing is out of alignment with who you are authentically. You may be guided to see the perfection of the problem. That is why my patients seek me out. They may not know this right away, but as we bring their body back into balance, they rediscover their true selves.

My wish for you is that every pain in your body and every unwanted situation in your life guides you and inspires you to discover and live your purpose. I hope that our paths cross again and that I may be of service to you in your journey.

Conclusion

Life does not always seem easy. Especially when you hit what looks like a low point. But I can guarantee you that, no matter how tough it may seem at the time, there is hope. In over a decade of working with people from all walks of life, and I mean all, I've helped thousands of them overcome their pain and discover the path to their authentic selves.

My Awareness, Awakening and Healing System, has been developed and refined over the years, not just from working with my patients, but through living and applying it myself. Overcoming cancer, obesity, impotence and high blood pressure at 26 was an eye opener for me and helped me to become the doctor I am today. After my pivotal trip to Thailand, that led to recreating myself, my life and my practice, my role in my patients health and lives jumped to a whole new level. I know that the evolution will only continue and I invite more lows so that I can get to ever new highs!

My wish for you, is that you are looking at your health, yourself and your life with a new set of eyes. That you are seeing the opportunity in your pain and symptoms and recognizing how symbolic the problems in your life can be.

I hope that you can look upon your life eagerly, with the knowledge that the right intentions and focus of your energy can change any pain, problem or situation into exactly what you want. This has certainly been my experience and that of thousands of people I've had the honor of working with.

The exercises and mindset shifts in this book have been included to help you see how much more you are than just your physical body and the massive impact that your thoughts and beliefs have on your health and life circumstances. I hope you are able to truly embrace your energetic nature and learn from the patterns that have been consistently showing up in your life. All of this is available to guide you in creating the life of your visions.

If I have gotten you to recognize, even a little, that you are being your own worst enemy when it comes to enjoying glowing health, happy and loving relationships and a life of joy, I am pleased. But if you feel that you would like to take what I have shared in this book to a deeper level in your life, I would be honored to guide you. I would love to be able to assist you in learning from your pain as you overcome it and change your beliefs around healing so you claim the limitless well-being that is rightfully yours. You will see, as so many of my patients have, that life truly is perfect and that you have power in shaping its perfection.

I invite you to email me at contact@drkeving.com to schedule a free consultation. There is always hope and we will be able to establish exactly what it will take to help you get the results you want. We will determine how we can

work together to move through the 5 Steps of my Awareness, Awakening and Healing System and get you the life
and health that you want.

Yours in gratitude,

Dr. Kevin

Appendix 1: Body Parts, Associated Emotions and Possible Symbolism

Body Part	Emotions/ Feelings	Possible Symbolism
Head - eyes, ears, nose, mouth	Perceptions	Your perspective vs. concern about others' perspective How you see the world, how things sound, concern about how things "smell", leaving a good or bad taste in your mouth.
Neck	Stubbornness, inflexibility	Refusing to see other sides of the question.
Throat	Communication	Concern for what was said, what should be said or what will be said.

Body Part	Emotions/ Feelings	Possible Symbolism
Shoulders	Responsibility	Carrying a burden Having difficulty accepting and living life in a joyous way.
Spine	Feeling supported	Upper- Feeling unloved. Mid - Guilt , stuck in the past, get off my back. Lower - Fear of money, lack of financial support.
Elbows	Acceptance of change	Changing directions and accepting new experiences.
Wrists	Freedom and ease	Feeling handcuffed to a situation. Being lead into an unwanted situation.
Hands	Attachment/ Control	Needing to get a hold of or get a grip on something. Hanging on too tightly Needing to let go.

Body Part	Emotions/ Feelings	Possible Symbolism
Hips	Fear of moving forward in decisions	Major decisions are necessary. Not having a focus to move forward towards.
Knees	Pride, ego, stubbornness	Inflexibility in life, unwillingness to bend, won't give in. Ego demanding its own way.
Ankles	Inflexibility and guilt	Trouble allowing self to receive pleasure.
Bunions	Lack of Joy	Not appreciating experiences in life.
Stomach	Sympathy/ Empathy	Not receiving proper resources for your intentions. Digesting an idea or experience. Finding a situation hard to digest.
Spleen	Sympathy/ Empathy	Needing to understand Embracing too much. Needing to clean up your act. Imbalance between lashing out and being to sweet.

Body Part	Emotions/ Feelings	Possible Symbolism
Lung	Guilt, grief, regret	Need for clarity and straightforwardness. Fear of speaking up. Stuck in grief or being too erratic.
Large Intestine	Sadness, grief, worry	Related to lungs. Holding things in
Kidney	Groaning, fears, anxiety	Needing to establish foundations.
Bladder	Jealousy, suspicion, grudges	Related to bladder. Indecision leading to diminishment of moral character.
Gallbladder	Anger, resentment, helplessness, choice	Needing to develop the courage and capacity to make decisions. Related to problems sleeping.
Liver	Transformation, resentment, bitterness, happiness	Ability to flow and spread. Feeling blocked. Stuck in toxic circumstances. Needing to refresh.

Body Part	Emotions/ Feelings	Possible Symbolism
Autonomic nervous system (Triple Warmer) and Endocrine system (Pericardium/ Circ-Sex)	Lightness, heaviness, hope, hysteria, balance, stubbornness, jealousy, exhaustion	Conflict between thoughts and emotions in daily activities. Needing to allow intuition and wisdom. Needing warmth. Life or death situations and causes worth fighting for.
Small Intestines	Excitement, joy, love, hate and laughter, Assimilation	Pure vs. impure. Needing nourishment. Needing encouragement.
Heart	Forgiveness, compassion, insecurity, self worth	Needing connection and circulation with your soul. Pride in legacy.

CPSIA information can be obtained
at www.ICGtesting.com
Printed in the USA
FFOW03n0110111217
43994281-43165FF

9 780998 854625